D1708829

The Achilles Tendon

The Achilles Tendon

Treatment and Rehabilitation

Edited by

James A. Nunley, MD

Duke University Medical Center, Durham, NC, USA

WITHDRAWN

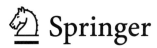 Springer

Editor
James A. Nunley
Duke University Medical Center
Department of Surgery
Division of Orthopaedic Surgery
Durham, NC 27110
USA
james.nunley@duke.edu

ISBN: 978-0-387-79205-7   e-ISBN: 978-0-387-79206-4
DOI: 10.1007/978-1-387-79206-4

Library of Congress Control Number: 2008930711

© Springer Science+Business Media, LLC 2009
All rights reserved. This work may not be translated or copied in whole or in part without the written permission of the publisher
(Springer Science+Business Media, LLC, 233 Spring Street, New York, NY 10013, USA), except for brief excerpts in connection
with reviews or scholarly analysis. Use in connection with any form of information storage and retrieval, electronic adaptation,
computer software, or by similar or dissimilar methodology now known or hereafter developed is forbidden.
The use in this publication of trade names, trademarks, service marks, and similar terms, even if they are not identified as such, is
not to be taken as an expression of opinion as to whether or not they are subject to proprietary rights.
While the advice and information in this book are believed to be true and accurate at the date of going to press, neither the authors
nor the editors nor the publisher can accept any legal responsibility for any errors or omissions that may be made. The publisher
makes no warranty, express or implied, with respect to the material contained herein.

Printed on acid-free paper

springer.com

To my wife, Elise,
for her love, support, and encouragement of so many years.

To my children, Ryan, Stephanie, and Jefferson,
for the excitement and joy that they have brought to my life.

To all of the residents and fellows at Duke University,
for their unwavering support and for providing me with intellectual
stimulation for so many years.

Foreword

Disorders of the Achilles tendon are universal, affecting people in a wide range of age groups. Because the Achilles tendon is one of the most powerful musculotendinous structures in the body, the impact of an injury to the Achilles tendon becomes magnified. There is a wide range of disorders or problems that can involve the insertional region, where pathology may rest with bone, tendon, or bursae. A completely different set of pathologic entities resides in the noninsertional region, one of which may include the frustrating degenerative tendinopathy. As our growing population ages but remains physically active longer into life, the incidence of these disorders will continue to increase.

I am proud to be given the opportunity to write the foreword to this text, which is intended for foot and ankle surgeons worldwide. Seldom does a book on a single entity become a current concepts review, as this work has. Too often, textbooks are not published for several years after the chapters have been written, making them obsolete upon publication. Not so with this book, which deals with timely topics on the Achilles tendon. Dr. James Nunley has compiled this work in slightly over a year, thus providing the reader with state-of-the-art material.

Dr. Nunley had the foresight to create a much needed techniques-oriented book dealing with the complexities of the Achilles tendon. His approach was to develop a comprehensive guide to managing Achilles tendon problems. You will learn not only the latest nonoperative approaches to specific Achilles problems, but also updated surgical techniques, with comparisons and references to traditional treatments. The chapters include a thorough description of indications and contraindications. Less invasive and minimally invasive technical advancements from the recent past are also included.

Dr. Nunley has met many experts in the field of foot and ankle surgery through his extensive travels and ongoing education in this subspecialty. He has enlisted these internationally renowned physicians to contribute chapters based on their vast experience. Introductory chapters provide essential background on basic anatomy, imaging, physiology, and pathomechanics, and subsequent sections cover the spectrum of Achilles tendon injuries. Acute and chronic conditions are addressed both in young adults and in elderly patients who are limited by Achilles symptoms. The book also takes a very practical approach to rehabilitation of the Achilles tendon postinjury and postsurgery. Athletic training, as it relates to the role of the Achilles complex, is highlighted with an emphasis on a faster return to play. Finally, case studies tie each chapter together and demonstrate the application of concepts to daily practice.

The text is further enhanced with high-definition photos and artwork, which include illustrated anatomy, MRIs, physical therapy tips, and surgical techniques and tools. Dr. Nunley has succeeded in compiling this information in a concise, understandable format.

I find this textbook to be extremely timely, given the complexities of the Achilles tendon and the large number of patients affected. This book will serve as a valuable reference—one that every orthopedic surgeon who manages such disorders will refer to often. I congratulate Dr. Nunley for the successful completion of this valuable endeavor.

February 5, 2008   Robert B. Anderson, MD

Preface

For many years, I participated in an instructional course lecture series for the American Academy of Orthopaedic Surgeons that addressed problems of the Achilles tendon. Through this lecture series it became apparent to me that there were numerous methods to treat the various pathologies associated with the Achilles tendon, but that there was no text available to guide surgeons in how to select the appropriate treatment. Thus, I felt that there was a need for a book to address not only historical issues associated with the Achilles tendon, but also the innovative ideas. A number of the authors of this text met at an international meeting where we discussed the possibility of a textbook. As we discussed a topic as simple as the weight-bearing status of a patient after an acute repair of the Achilles tendon, I saw that there was a wide and diverse group of opinions among the experts. This textbook consolidates these opinions to help guide students, patients, therapists, and surgeons in deciding on a course of treatment.

I have had many friends ask why a topic as simple as the Achilles tendon requires a textbook. I think the reader will agree that the amount of information available today concerning injury and repair of the Achilles justifies a textbook dedicated to the topic. The book addresses the anatomy and imaging characteristics of the Achilles tendon, as well as the assessment of acute and chronic injuries, which over the years has seen numerous refinements in surgical technique for repair and rehabilitation. The last section of the book addresses chronic tendinopathy, which is a vast area and incorporates many degenerative and athletic injuries.

The chapters in this text were written by experts who have been recognized worldwide for their contributions. The text presents the most common surgical procedure for any given condition, as well as any debate that might still exist. This text can help practitioners decide if they should treat the acute rupture of the Achilles tendon nonoperatively or with a percutaneous technique, with a mini-open procedure or with a formal open repair. The text also discusses the pros, cons, risks, and benefits of each of these surgical techniques. A case-based example in each chapter helps provide the reader with a greater understanding of the possible solutions available for any given problem.

My hope is that this text will provide a stimulus for the improved treatment of the many types of injuries to the Achilles, and guidance for those who are in the trenches treating the pathologies relating to Achilles tendon disorders.

February 7, 2008   James A. Nunley, MD

Contents

Contributors

Robert B. Anderson, MD, BS
OrthoCarolina Foot and Ankle Institute, 1001 Blythe Boulevard, Suite 200,
Charlotte, NC 28203, USA

Mathieu Assal, MD
Médecin Adjoint du Chef de Service, FMH Chirurgie Orthopédic et de
Traumatologie de l'appareil moteur, Hôpitaux Universitaires de Genève,
Rue Micheli-du-Crest 24, CH-1211 Genève 14, Switzerland

Christoph Becher, MD
Department of Orthopaedics, Hannover Medical School, Anna-von-Borries-
Str. 1-7, 30625 Hannover, Germany

W. Hodges Davis, MD
Department of Orthopaedics, Hannover Medical School, Anna-von-
Borries-Str. 1-7, 30625 Hannover, Germany

Andrew M. Ebert, MD, BA
Orthopaedic Specialists of Austin, 1015 East 32nd Street, Suite 505,
Austin, Texas 78705, USA

Mark E. Easley, MD
Duke University Medical Center, Division of Orthopaedic Surgery, Duke
Health Center, 3115 North Duke Street, Rm 243, Durham, NC 27704, USA

William E. Garrett Jr., MD, PhD
Professor, Division of Orthopaedic Surgery, Box 3338, Duke University
Medical Center, Durham, NC 27710, USA

Clyde A. Helms, MD
Division Chief, Musculoskeletal Radiology, Duke University Medical Center,
Department of Radiology, Box 3808, Durham, NC 27710, USA

Beat Hintermann, MD
Associate Professor, University of Basel, Clinic of Orthopaedics, Kantonsspital,
Rheinstrasse, Liestal CH-4410, Switzerland

Anish R. Kadakia, MD
Institute for Foot and Ankle Reconstruction, Mercy Medical Center, 301
Saint Paul Place, Baltimore, MD 21202, USA

Maria Kyriaki Kaseta, MD
Fellow, Sports Medicine, Duke University, Department of Surgery,
280 Frank Bassett Drive, Durham, NC 27708, USA

Markus Knupp, MD
Senior attending resident, Clinic of Orthopaedics, Rheinstrasse, Liestal
CH-4410, Switzerland

Ian L. D. Le, MD, FRCS(C)
Clinical Lecturer, University of Calgary, Peter Lougheed Hospital,
Department of Surgery, Division of Orthopaedics 2675 36st NE, Calgary,
Alberta, T1Y 6H6, Canada

L. Scott Levin, MD
Chief, Division of Plastic and Reconstructive Surgery, Duke University
Medical Center, Durham, NC 27710, USA

Nicola Maffulli, MD, MS, PhD, FRCS (Orth)
Professor, Keele University School of Medicine, Department of Trauma and
Orthopaedic Surgery, Stoke-on-Trent, Staffordshire ST4 7QB, UK

Ansar Mahmood, MB ChB, MRCS (Edinburgh)
Specialist Registrar, Leighton Hospital, Trauma and Orthopaedics,
Middlewich Road, Crewe, Cheshire, CW1 4QJ, UK

Claude T. Moorman III, MD
Associate Professor, Director, Sports Medicine, Duke University Medical
Center, Department of Orthopaedic Surgery, 311 Finch Yeager Building,
Frank Bassett Drive, Durham, NC 27708, USA

Kurtis Moyer, MD
Plastic Surgery Resident, Division of Plastic and Reconstructive Surgery,
Duke University Medical Center, Durham, NC 27710, USA

George A. C. Murrell, MD, PhD
Professor, University of New South Wales, St. George Hospital Campus,
Department of Orthopaedic Surgery, Level 2, 4-10 South Street, Kogarah,
Sydney, New South Wales, 2217, Australia

Mark S. Myerson, MD
Director, Institute for Foot and Ankle Reconstruction, Mercy Medical Center,
301 Saint Paul Place, Baltimore, MD 21202, USA

Florian Nickisch, MD
Assistant Professor of Orthopaedics, University of Utah Orthopaedic Center,
590 Wakara Way, Salt Lake City, UT 84108 USA

James A. Nunley, MD
Goldner-Jones Professor and Chief of Orthopaedics, Duke University
Medical Center, Box 2923 DUMC, Durham, NC 27710, USA

Justin A. Paoloni, MBBS, BSc (med), PhD, MspMed, FACSP
Sports Physician, University of New South Wales, Orthopaedic Research
Institute, Research and Education Center, 2nd Floor, 4-10 South Street,
Kogaram, New South Wales, 2217, Australia

John S. Reach Jr., MSc, MD
Director, Foot & Ankle Service, Yale University School of Medicine,
Department of Orthopaedic Surgery & Rehabilitation, Yale Physicians
Building 113, 800 Howard Ave., New Haven, CT 06520-8071, USA

Kush Singh, MD
Musculoskeletal Fellow, Duke University Medical Center, Department
of Radiology, Box 3808, Durham, NC 27710, USA

Hajo Thermann, MD, PhD
Atos-Clinic Center, Heidelberg, Center for Knee and Foot Surgery,
Bismarckstrasse 9-15, Heidelberg 69115, Germany

Troy S. Watson, MD
Director, Foot and Ankle Institute, Desert Orthopaedic Center,
2880 East Desert Inn Road, Suite 100, Las Vegas, NV 89121, USA

Joseph Yu, MD
Nevada Orthopedic and Spine Center, Department of Orthopaedics,
2650 North Tenaya Way, Suite 301, Las Vegas, NV 89183, USA

Section I

Introduction

1

Anatomy of the Achilles Tendon

Florian Nickisch

The Achilles tendon is the conjoined tendon of the two heads of the gastrocnemius and the soleus muscle. Together these structures are often referred to as the "gastroc-soleus complex." It is the largest and strongest tendon in the human body and subject to tensile forces of up to 12.5 times body weight (9 kilonewton [kN]) during sprinting[1] and six to eight times body weight during athletic activity such as jumping or cycling.[2] Due to its size and functional demands, the Achilles tendon is susceptible to both acute and chronic injuries and is directly or indirectly implicated in many pathologic conditions of the foot and ankle. To diagnose and treat these disorders, a thorough knowledge of the anatomy of the Achilles tendon and its surrounding structures is crucial.

Microstructure

Tendons are complex, composite, roughly uniaxial structures consisting of collagen fibrils embedded in a matrix, rich in water and proteoglycans with a paucity of cells. Collagen (mainly type I collagen) accounts for 65% to 80%, and elastin for approximately 2%, of the dry mass of the tendon. The predominant cells are tenoblasts and tenocytes (elongated fibroblasts). Their spindle-shaped cell bodies are arranged in rows between the collagen fiber bundles and they produce the extracellular matrix proteins. Soluble tropocollagen molecules are cross-linked to create insoluble collagen molecules, which then aggregate into microfibrils. Further aggregation leads to the formation of collagen fibrils. The diameter of collagen fibrils in the Achilles tendon varies from 30 nm to 150 nm.[3] The basic unit of a tendon, the collagen fiber, is created by the binding of multiple collagen fibrils (Fig. 1.1). Each collagen fiber is surrounded by a fine sheath of connective tissue, the endotenon, which allows the fiber groups to glide and provides access channels for blood vessels, nerves, and lymphatics to the deep portions of the tendon. Moreover, the endotenon binds fibers together to form primary fiber bundles (subfascicles), which then group to form secondary fiber bundles or fascicles. A group of secondary bundles then forms the tertiary bundle, with an average diameter of 1000 to 3000 μm through incorporation in a proteoglycan-rich extracellular matrix.[4]

J.A. Nunley (ed.), *The Achilles Tendon: Treatment and Rehabilitation*,
DOI: 10.1007/978-1-387-79206-4_1, © Springer Science+Business Media, LLC 2009

3

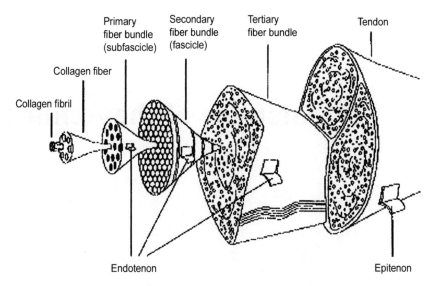

Fig. 1.1. The organization of tendon structure from collagen fibrils to the entire tendon. (From Kannus,[4] with permission from Blackwell Publishing.)

The tendon is made up of several tertiary bundles surrounded by the epitenon. On its outer surface, the epitenon is in contact with the paratenon, whereas the inner surface the epitenon is continuous with the endotenon,[1]

Gross Anatomy

The leg consists of four compartments (anterior, lateral, superficial, and deep posterior) divided by strong fascial septa. The superficial posterior compartment contains the gastroc-soleus complex and the plantaris muscle, supplied by the tibial nerve and branches from the posterior tibial and peroneal arteries. It is separated from the deep posterior compartment by the deep leaf of the fascia cruris.

Gastrocnemius

The gastrocnemius muscle crosses the knee, ankle, and subtalar joint; hence, it is maximally stretched with the knee fully extended and the ankle dorsiflexed while the heel is inverted.[5] Consisting mainly of fast twitch muscle fibers, the gastrocnemius muscle flexes the knee, plantar flexes the ankle, and inverts the subtalar joint. It is the most superficial muscle in the calf and is responsible for its contour. The two heads of the gastrocnemius muscle are firmly attached to the posterior aspect of the femur, just proximal to the femoral condyles, by strong, flat tendons that expand into a short aponeurosis on the posterior surface of the muscle bellies. Both heads also attach to the posterior aspect of the knee joint capsule onto the oblique popliteal ligament. The medial, larger head takes its origin slightly superior to the lateral head and extends more distal in the calf (Fig. 1.2). Deep to the medial head is usually a bursa that often communicates with the knee joint. In 10% to 30% of the population, there is a sesamoid bone (fabella) in the proximal tendon of the lateral head of the gastrocnemius that often directly articulates with the lateral femoral condyle.[6]

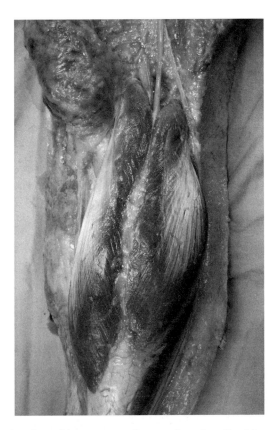

Fig. 1.2. Posterior view of the gastrocnemius muscle and popliteal fossa. The common peroneal nerve passes just lateral to the lateral head, whereas the tibial neurovascular bundle passes between the medial and lateral heads of the muscle

When present, it is usually bilateral and serves as an attachment site for the fabellofibular ligament in the posterolateral corner of the knee joint capsule. The muscle fibers from each head run obliquely and attach at an angle in the middle of the calf into a midline raphe that further distal broadens into an aponeurosis on the anterior surface of the muscle. This aponeurosis gradually narrows and unites with the tendon of the soleus to form the Achilles tendon. The gastrocnemius is innervated by the first and second sacral roots through the tibial nerve.

Soleus

The soleus is a postural muscle consisting mainly of slow-twitch muscle fibers. It helps to keep the body upright in stance and prevents the body from falling forward during gait, as it contracts when the center of gravity passes in front of the knee joint. It is the strongest muscle in the lower leg and the prime plantar flexor of the ankle joint.[7] The soleus has its origin on the posterior surface of the fibula head and the proximal 25% of the posterior surface of the fibula as well as the middle third of the posteromedial border of the tibia. Some fibers arise from the fibrous arch between the tibial and fibular origins of the muscle. The soleus is a pennate muscle. It is wider than the gastrocnemius and consists of an anterior and a posterior aponeurosis with the bulk of the muscle fibers in between (Fig. 1.3). The muscle architecture is nonuniform with variable fiber lengths between 16 and 45 mm.[8] The muscle fibers extend more distally than those of the gastrocnemius and insert into the posterior aponeurosis, which lies directly anterior to the aponeurosis of the gastrocnemius. The two aponeurotic leafs of the soleus lie parallel for a variable distance before they join in the distal lower leg prior to uniting with the tendon of the gastrocnemius to form the Achilles tendon. Usually the soleus tendon contributes more fibers to the Achilles tendon than the gastrocnemius.[7] The gastrocnemius is innervated by the first and second sacral roots through the tibial nerve.

An accessory soleus muscle has been recognized since the 19th century. Originally thought to be a rare finding, it has been diagnosed more frequently since the introduction of magnetic resonance imaging (MRI) into clinical practice.[9] The reported incidence ranges from 0.7% to 6%.[10–12] Its presence may be accounted for by the splitting of the anlage of the soleus early in development and may be unilateral or bilateral.[13] The proximal origin is typically on the distal posterior aspect of the tibia, and less commonly on the deep fascia of the normal soleus or other flexor tendons.[10,12] The accessory soleus most commonly inserts via a separate tendon on the calcaneus, anteromedial to

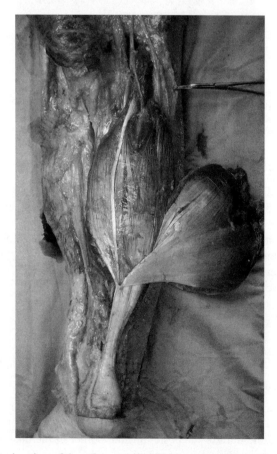

Fig. 1.3. Posterior view of the soleus muscle. The gastrocnemius has been detached at its origin and reflected laterally, exposing the plantaris muscle and tendon

the Achilles tendon insertion. Other insertions include those on the Achilles tendon, superior calcaneus, or lateral calcaneus.[11] The anomalous muscle is usually enclosed in its own fascia and has its own blood supply via branches from the posterior tibial artery. The presence of an accessory soleus muscle is clinically relevant as it may be a source of posteromedial ankle pain, likely related to a localized, exertional compartment syndrome.[11]

Plantaris

The plantaris has it origin on the lower part of the lateral prolongation of the linea aspera, and on the oblique popliteal ligament of the posterolateral knee joint capsule. It has a small fusiform, usually a 7- to 10-cm-long muscle belly. The thin plantaris tendon crosses obliquely between the gastrocnemius and soleus muscles and then runs parallel to the medial aspect of the Achilles tendon (Fig. 1.3). It inserts most commonly into the posteromedial part of the calcaneal tuberosity.[14] Occasionally, the tendon is lost in the laciniate ligament or in the fascia of the leg. The plantaris is absent in 6% to 8% of individuals.

Achilles Tendon

The Achilles tendon originates in the middle of the lower leg as the confluence of the tendons of the gastrocnemius and soleus muscles at the gastroc-soleus junction (Figs. 1.3 and 1.4). The length of the conjoined tendon is approximately 10 to 15 cm, that of the gastrocnemius component ranges from 11 to 26 cm, and that of the soleus component ranges from 3 to 11 cm.[14] The thickness of the Achilles tendon was measured with ultrasonography and MRI in 267 healthy individuals of various ages. Children under 10 had a tendon thickness (mean ± standard deviation [SD]) of 4.6 ± 0.8 mm, 10 to 17 years of age 6.1 ± 0.8 mm, 18 to 30 years of age 6.3 ± 0.5 mm, and over 30 years of age 6.9 ± 1.0 mm.[15] The distance from the most distal extent of the gastrocnemius muscle fibers to the gastroc-soleus junction varies from 2 to 8 cm.[16]

Muscle fibers of the soleus may insert into the anterior surface of the tendon to almost its insertion. The contribution of fibers of the gastrocnemius and soleus to the Achilles tendon is variable. In most individuals, the soleus contributes more fibers than the gastrocnemius, as demonstrated by Cummins and coworkers[14] in anatomic dissections of 100 specimens. At the gastroc-soleus junction, the Achilles tendon is broad and flat. As it travels distally in the leg, it becomes progressively ovoid in cross section, to a level 4 cm proximal to its insertion, where it can become relatively flatter again.[14] During their descent, the fibers of the Achilles tendon internally rotate to a variable degree (approximately 90 degrees) in a spiral manner,[17] so that the initially posterior fibers of the soleus insert mainly on the medial aspect of the Achilles tendon footprint, whereas those of the gastrocnemius (initially anterior) insert laterally. The extent of fiber rotation is determined by the position of fusion between the two muscles, with a more distal fusion resulting in more rotation. This rotation makes elongation and elastic recoil within the tendon possible and allows the release of stored energy during the appropriate phase of gait.[18,19] This stored energy allows the generation of higher shortening velocities and greater instantaneous muscle power than could be achieved by contraction of the gastrocnemius and soleus muscles alone.[18,19] Fiber rotation reaches a maximum 2 to 5 cm proximal to the tendon insertion and creates high stresses in this

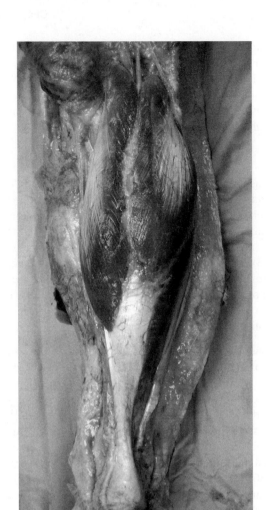

Fig. 1.4. Posterior view of the Achilles tendon

area of the tendon, which may explain the poor vascularity and susceptibility to degeneration and injury in this region.

The Achilles tendon inserts on the middle third of the posterior surface of the calcaneal tuberosity, starting approximately 1 cm distal to the most superior border of the bone (Fig. 1.5).[20] The average area of insertion is approximately 19.8 mm in length with a width of 24 mm proximally and 31 mm distally.[20,21] Typically the distance of insertion is longer on the medial side.[20] More distally the tendon fibers transition into the periosteum of the calcaneus. In neonates there is a continuous heavy layer of collagen fibers connecting the Achilles tendon and the plantar fascia; however, the number of these fibers decreases with age and they eventually disappear completely.[22]

The attachment site of the Achilles tendon displays the typical structure of a fibrocartilaginous enthesis, and thus four zones of tissue are commonly present: pure dense fibrous connective tissue, uncalcified fibrocartilage, calcified fibrocartilage, and bone (Fig. 1.6).[23,24] The zones of uncalcified and

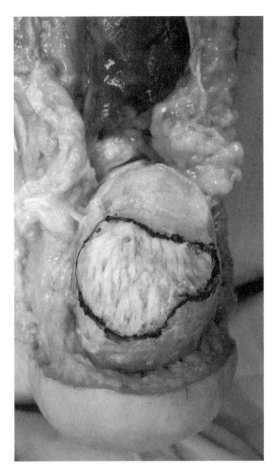

Fig. 1.5. Achilles tendon insertion on the posterior aspect of the calcaneal tuberosity. Note the broader area of insertion on the medial aspect as well as its central location on the calcaneal tuberosity

calcified fibrocartilage at the osteotendinous junction are referred to as the enthesis fibrocartilage. It dissipates the bending of tendon fibers away from the hard tissue interface and thereby protects them.[25]

Directly anterior to the tendon insertion, between the posterior surface of the calcaneus and the Achilles tendon, is the retrocalcaneal bursa (Fig. 1.7). The bursa is a wedge-shaped sac that is horseshoe-shaped in cross section with arms extending on the medial and lateral edge of the tendon. It mainly consists of synovial projections that allow alteration in its shape with plantarflexion and dorsiflexion of the ankle to promote free movement between tendon and bone.[26] The posterior wall of the bursa, however, is made up of sesamoid fibrocartilage on the anterior surface of the Achilles tendon.[27] This sesamoid fibrocartilage enables the tendon to resist compressive loading where it "articulates" with a corresponding periosteal fibrocartilage on the posterosuperior calcaneus (the anterior wall of the bursa) during dorsiflexion of the foot.[27] The enthesis and the periosteal fibrocartilage can be viewed as a series of pulleys that provide the Achilles tendon with an efficient moment arm[28] and mechanical advantage in its action on the calcaneus (Fig. 1.8).

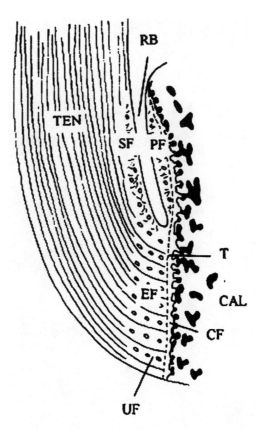

Fig. 1.6. A diagrammatic representation of the attachment of the human Achilles tendon (TEN) to the calcaneus (CAL). Note the three fibrocartilages at the insertion site: Enthesial fibrocartilage (EF) at the bone–tendon junction; sesamoid fibrocartilage (SF) on the adjacent, deep surface of the tendon; and periosteal fibrocartilage (PF) on the opposing surface of the calcaneus. SF and PF are separated by the retrocalcaneal bursa (RF), but they are pressed against each other during ankle movements. EF has a zone of uncalcified fibrocartilage (UF), which is separated from a zone of calcified fibrocartilage (CF) by a tidemark (T), indicated by the broken line. (From Waggett et al.,[24] with permission from Elsevier.)

The space between the Achilles tendon and the posterior border of the tibia is known as Kager's triangle. It is occupied by a mass of adipose tissue: Kager's fat pad. This fat pad consists of three distinct regions: the superficial Achilles-associated part, the deep flexor hallucis longus (FHL)-associated part, and a calcaneal bursal wedge, which moves into the bursa during plantar-flexion.[29] The mechanical functions of the fat pad include reducing friction between the tendon and the bone, preventing the tendon from kinking under load, acting as a variable space filler to prevent buildup of negative pressure in the bursa during plantarflexion, and protecting blood vessels supplying the tendon.[23,29] It may also play a role in proprioception, as it contains a variety of sensory nerve endings.[30]

The Achilles tendon is an extrasynovial tendon without a true synovial tendon sheath. Throughout its length the tendon is surrounded by the paratenon, a thin gliding membrane of loose areolar tissue, that permits free movement of

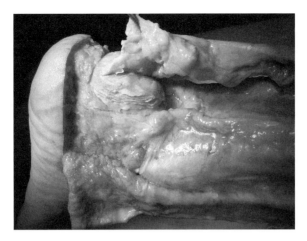

Fig. 1.7. Lateral view of the Achilles tendon insertion. The tendon has been partially reflected off the calcaneus exposing the retrocalcaneal bursa

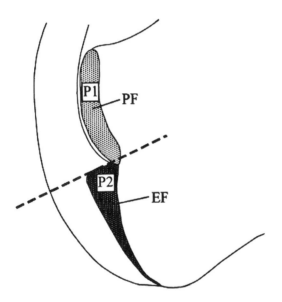

Fig. 1.8. A diagrammatic representation of how the periosteal (PF) and enthesis (EF) fibrocartilages could be viewed as two pulleys (P1 and P2) in series with each other, to increase the moment arm of the Achilles tendon at its insertion. The periosteal fibrocartilage, covering the superior tuberosity of the calcaneus, acts as a pulley for the Achilles tendon above the level of the broken line (P1), altering the direction of its collagen fibers. Below the line, the enthesis fibrocartilage acts as a pulley at the insertion site itself (P2). (From Milz et al.,[28] with permission from Blackwell Publishing.)

the tendon within the surrounding tissues, and, although not as effectively as a true tendon sheath, significantly reduces the gliding resistance of the tendon (Fig. 1.9).[31] Under the paratenon, the entire Achilles tendon is surrounded by a fine, smooth connective tissue sheath called the epitenon. On its outer surface, the epitenon is in contact with the paratenon. The inner surface of the epitenon

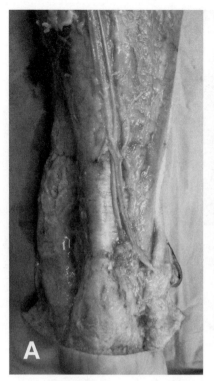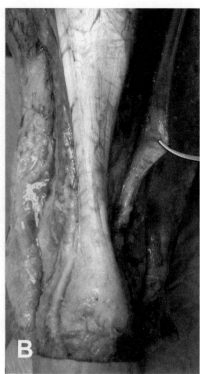

Fig. 1.9. (A) Posterior view of the soft tissues surrounding the Achilles tendon. Note the course of the sural nerve and lesser saphenous vein as they cross the lateral border of the tendon. (B) The paratenon has been reflected, exposing the Achilles tendon

is continuous with the endotenon, which binds the collagen fibers and fiber bundles together and provides neural, vascular, and lymphatic access channels to the tendon.[1]

Vascularity of the Achilles Tendon

The Achilles tendon receives its blood supply from three main sources: the intrinsic vascular systems at the myotendinous junction and the osteotendinous junction, and from the extrinsic segmental vascular system through the paratenon surrounding the tendon.[1] At the myotendinous junction, blood vessels from the muscle bellies penetrate the endotenon and contribute to the blood supply of the proximal third of the tendon. This contribution, however, is thought to be less significant, as only the vessels in the perimysium continue on to the tendon.[32–34] The majority of the Achilles tendon is vascularized throughout its length by branches of the posterior tibial artery in the paratenon on the anterior surface of the tendon. These vessels reach the tendon through a series of transverse vincula, enter the tendon substance along the endotenon, and then run parallel to the axis of the tendon. The proximal part of the tendon receives additional blood supply through a recurrent branch of the posterior tibial artery, whereas distally the rete arteriosum calcaneum formed by branches of the posterior tibial, peroneal, and lateral plantar arteries,

Table 1.1 Summary of studies reporting regions of human achilles tendon vascularization.

	Technique	Result Most vascularization	Least vascularization
Ahmed et al.	Histologic blood vessel density-quantitative study	Insertion	Midsection and origin
Astrom	Qualitative laser Doppler flowmetry study	Midsection and origin	Insertion
Astrom and Westlin	Quantitative laser Doppler flowmetry study	Midsection and origin	Insertion
Carr and Norris	Angiographic qualitative study (of vessels greater than 20 μm in diameter)	Insertion	Midsection
Lagergren and Lindholm	Angiographic qualitative study	Origin and insertion	Midsection
Langberg et al.	Radioisotope tracking of tendon blood flow-quantitative study	Midsection	Insertion
Schmidt-Rohlfing et al.	Epoxy resin injections highlighting vessels-qualitative study	Midsection	Insertion
Silvestri et al.	Qualitative power Doppler study	No flow recorded	No flow recorded
Stein et al.	Quantitative intravascular volume	Origin	Midsection
Zantop et al.	Immunohistochemical quantitative vascular density study	Origin	Midsection

From Theobald et al.,[36] with permission from Elsevier.

contributes significantly to the vascularization of the tendon.[35] The distribution of vascularity throughout the Achilles tendon is not homogeneous.[36–41] Despite varying reports, the majority of authors on the subject believe that the blood supply to the midsection of the tendon is the poorest, with an area of lowest vascularity approximately 2 to 6 cm proximal to the tendon insertion (Table 1.1) As this area of relative hypovascularity correlates with the most common site of rupture of the Achilles tendon, it is believed that the lack of blood supply either directly decreases the tensile strength[42,43] or indirectly weakens the tendon through degenerative changes.[34,44]

Innervation of the Achilles Tendon

The Achilles tendon is supplied by nerves from the attaching muscles and by small fasciculi from cutaneous nerves, in particular the sural nerve.[45] The sural nerve is a purely sensory nerve, formed by the confluence of the medial cutaneous branch of the tibial nerve and the peroneal communicating branch off the lateral sural cutaneous nerve emanating from the common peroneal nerve. It descends distally between the heads of the gastrocnemius and takes a highly variable course. At the level of the gastroc-soleus junction, the sural nerve lies approximately 46 mm (range, 27 to 69 mm) lateral to the medial border of the gastrocnemius tendon,[46] or 12 mm (range, 7 to 17 mm) medial to the lateral border.[47] At this level it may be superficial or deep to the muscle fascia.[46] When performing a gastrocnemius recession (Strayer procedure), the sural nerve is especially at risk, as it has been shown to be directly applied to the gastrocnemius tendon in approximately 10%.[46] The sural nerve crosses the lateral border of the Achilles tendon an average of 9.83 cm (range, 6.5 to 16 cm) proximal to the tendon insertion[48] and then courses anteriorly towards the lateral border of the foot (Fig. 1.9A). Small branches of the sural nerve form the longitudinal plexus and enter the tendon through the endotenon. Some also pass from the paratenon by way of the epitenon to reach the surface or the interior of the tendon (Fig. 1.9B).[49] The number of nerves and nerve endings is relatively low in large tendons such as the Achilles, and many nerve fibers terminate on the tendon surface or in the paratenon. Nevertheless, the Achilles tendon contains numerous receptors relating to both pain and other neurotransmitter actions.[1,30]

References

1. Paavola M, Kannus P, Jarvinen TA, et al. Achilles tendinopathy. J Bone Joint Surg [Am] 2002;84A:2062–76.
2. Soma CA, Mandelbaum BR. Achilles tendon disorders. Clin Sports Med 1994;13:811–23.
3. Magnusson SP, Qvortrup K, Larsen JO, et al. Collagen fibril size and crimp morphology in ruptured and intact Achilles tendons. Matrix Biol 2002;21:369–77.
4. Kannus P. Structure of the tendon connective tissue. Scand J Med Sci Sports 2000;10:312–20.
5. DiGiovanni CW, Kuo R, Tejwani N, et al. Isolated gastrocnemius tightness. J Bone Joint Surg [Am] 2002;84A:962–70.
6. Duncan W, Dahm DL. Clinical anatomy of the fabella. Clin Anat 2003;16:448–9.
7. Kvist M. Achilles tendon injuries in athletes. Sports Med 1994;18:173–201.
8. Agur AM, Ng-Thow-Hing V, Ball KA, et al. Documentation and three-dimensional modeling of human soleus muscle architecture. Clin Anat 2003;16:285–93.
9. Apple JS MS, Khoury MB, Nunley JA. Case report 376. Skeletal Radiol 1986;15:398–400.
10. Agur AM, McKee N, Leekam R. Accessory soleus muscle, American Association of Clinical Anatomists Meeting, Honolulu, Hawaii, 1997.
11. Brodie JT, Dormans JP, Gregg JR, et al. Accessory soleus muscle. A report of 4 cases and review of literature. Clin Orthop Rel Res 1997:180–6.
12. Palaniappan M, Rajesh A, Rickett A, et al. Accessory soleus muscle: a case report and review of the literature. Pediatr Radiol 1999;29:610–2.
13. Gordon SL, Matheson D. The accessory soleus. Clin Orthop Rel Res 1973;97:129–137.
14. Cummins EJA, Anderson BJ, Carr BW, Wright RR. The structure of the calcaneal tendon (of Achilles) in relation to orthopaedic surgery. With additional observations on the plantaris muscle. Surg Gynecol Obstet 1946;83:107–116.
15. Koivunen-Niemela T, Parkkola K. Anatomy of the Achilles tendon (tendo calcaneus) with respect to tendon thickness measurements. Surg Radiol Anat 1995;17:263–8.
16. Carl T BSL. Cadaveric assessment of the gastrocnemius aponeurosis to assist in the pre-operative planning for two-portal endoscopic gastrocnemius recession (EGR). Foot 2005;15:137–140.
17. Sarrafian S. Anatomy of the Foot and Ankle. Philadelphia: JB Lippincott, 1993.
18. Alexander RM, Bennet-Clark HC. Storage of elastic strain energy in muscle and other tissues. Nature 1977;265:114–117.
19. Maffulli N. Rupture of the Achilles tendon. J Bone Joint Surg [Am] 1999;81:1019–36.

20. Chao W, Deland JT, Bates JE, et al. Achilles tendon insertion: an in vitro anatomic study. Foot Ankle Int 1997;18:81–4.
21. Kolodziej P, Glisson RR, Nunley JA. Risk of avulsion of the Achilles tendon after partial excision for treatment of insertional tendonitis and Haglund's deformity: a biomechanical study. Foot Ankle Int 1999;20:433–7.
22. Snow SW, Bohne WH, DiCarlo E, et al. Anatomy of the Achilles tendon and plantar fascia in relation to the calcaneus in various age groups. Foot Ankle Int 1995;16:418–21.
23. Benjamin M, Toumi H, Ralphs JR, et al. Where tendons and ligaments meet bone: attachment sites ('entheses') in relation to exercise and/or mechanical load. J Anat 2006;208:471–90.
24. Waggett AD, Ralphs JR, Kwan AP, et al. Characterization of collagens and proteoglycans at the insertion of the human Achilles tendon. Matrix Biol 1998;16:457–70.
25. Benjamin M, Ralphs JR. Fibrocartilage in tendons and ligaments—an adaptation to compressive load. J Anat 1998;193(pt 4):481–94.
26. Canoso JJ, Liu N, Traill MR, et al. Physiology of the retrocalcaneal bursa. Ann Rheum Dis 1988;47:910–2.
27. Rufai A, Ralphs JR, Benjamin M. Structure and histopathology of the insertional region of the human Achilles tendon. J Orthop Res 1995;13:585–93.
28. Milz S, Rufai A, Buettner A, et al. Three-dimensional reconstructions of the Achilles tendon insertion in man. J Anat 2002;200:145–52.
29. Theobald P, Bydder G, Dent C, et al. The functional anatomy of Kager's fat pad in relation to retrocalcaneal problems and other hindfoot disorders. J Anat 2006;208:91–7.
30. Bjur D, Alfredson H, Forsgren S. The innervation pattern of the human Achilles tendon: studies of the normal and tendinosis tendon with markers for general and sensory innervation. Cell Tissue Res 2005;320:201–6.
31. Momose T AP, Zobitz ME, Zhao C, et al. Effect of paratenon and repetitive motion on the gliding resistance of tendon of extrasynovial origin. Clin Anat 2002;15:199-205.
32. Kvist M, Hurme T, Kannus P, et al. Vascular density at the myotendinous junction of the rat gastrocnemius muscle after immobilization and remobilization. Am J Sports Med 1995;23:359–64.
33. Ahmed IM, Lagopoulos M, McConnell P, et al. Blood supply of the Achilles tendon. J Orthop Res 1998;16:591–6.
34. Langberg H, Bulow J, Kjaer M. Blood flow in the peritendinous space of the human Achilles tendon during exercise. Acta Physiol Scand 1998;163:149–53.
35. Sanz-Hospital FJ, Martin CM, Escalera J, et al. Achilleo-calcaneal vascular network. Foot Ankle Int 1997;18:506–9.
36. Theobald P, Benjamin M, Nokes L, et al. Review of the vascularisation of the human Achilles tendon. Injury 2005;36:1267–72.
37. Astrom M, Westlin N. Blood flow in the human Achilles tendon assessed by laser Doppler flowmetry. J Orthop Res 1994;12:246–52.
38. Astrom M. Laser Doppler flowmetry in the assessment of tendon blood flow. Scand J Med Sci Sports 2000;10:365–7.
39. Carr AJ, Norris SH. The blood supply of the calcaneal tendon. J Bone Joint Surg Br 1989;71:100–1.
40. Silvestri E, Biggi E, Molfetta L, et al. Power Doppler analysis of tendon vascularization. Int J Tissue React 2003;25:149–58.
41. Stein V, Laprell H, Tinnemeyer S, et al. Quantitative assessment of intravascular volume of the human Achilles tendon. Acta Orthop Scand 2000;71:60–3.
42. Lagergren C, Lindholm A. Vascular distribution in the Achilles tendon; an angiographic and microangiographic study. Acta Chir Scand 1959;116:491–5.

43. Schmidt-Rohlfing B, Graf J, Schneider U, et al. The blood supply of the Achilles tendon. Int Orthop 1992;16:29–31.
44. Zantop T, Tillmann B, Petersen W. Quantitative assessment of blood vessels of the human Achilles tendon: an immunohistochemical cadaver study. Arch Orthop Trauma Surg 2003;123:501–4.
45. Stilwell DL Jr. The innervation of tendons and aponeuroses. Am J Anat 1957;100:289–317.
46. Pinney SJ, Sangeorzan BJ, Hansen ST Jr. Surgical anatomy of the gastrocnemius recession (Strayer procedure). Foot Ankle Int 2004;25:247–50.
47. Tashjian RZ, Appel AJ, Banerjee R, et al. Anatomic study of the gastrocnemius-soleus junction and its relationship to the sural nerve. Foot Ankle Int 2003;24:473–6.
48. Webb J, Moorjani N, Radford M. Anatomy of the sural nerve and its relation to the Achilles tendon. Foot Ankle Int 2000;21:475–7.
49. Josza G, Kannus P. Human Tendons: Anatomy, Physiology, and Pathology Human Kinetics, 1997 Leeds, UK.

2

Ultrasound Examination of the Achilles Tendon

John S. Reach, Jr. and James A. Nunley

There is growing evidence that the clinical and operative use of ultrasound imaging can benefit patients with Achilles tendon pathology. Although ultrasonography has been stigmatized as too operator dependent and necessitating a steep learning curve, it has been our experience that the modality is relatively straightforward. Surgeons are in a unique position to utilize this technology, as they have the firm grasp of anatomy that is essential to the interpretation of sonograms. Ultrasound provides real-time dynamic imaging in the office and in the operative setting that directly benefits our patients. Ultrasound images can assist the clinician in determining the exact pathologic process, including location of symptoms, assessment of concurrent pathology, response to treatment, and the planning and intraoperative assessment of tendinous pathology.

The Achilles tendon is the largest superficially located tendon of the body and is ideally suited to ultrasound examination. Achilles tendon morphology is best visualized with a high-frequency linear transducer (5 to 10 MHz).

After an appropriate history and physical is obtained, the patient is positioned prone with both lower extremities disrobed (Fig. 2.1). As with all tendons, images of the Achilles tendon should be obtained in two orthogonal planes. Longitudinal and transverse images should be obtained from the musculotendinous junction to the distal tendon insertion on the calcaneus.

To obtain an orderly and reproducible examination, imaging begins directly over the area of pain or tenderness with the foot in the gravity neutral position. In general, transverse imaging is followed by longitudinal imaging. Because ultrasound is a dynamic imaging modality, movie clips of the examination can be saved in the patient's electronic record. After the static examination of the area of interest, the surgeon grasps the patient's foot, introducing passive dorsiflexion and plantarflexion. This is followed by visualization of the symptomatic area with active range of motion. Finally, a full examination of the tendon from its most distal insertion proximally to the myotendinous junction is performed. Obviously, examination may be extended to the gastrocnemius and soleus muscles, depending on the clinical situation.

The normal Achilles tendon, as shown in Figure 2.2, appears echogenic (bright) with an organized fibrillar ultrastructure. The paratenon envelops the tendon as a thin, echogenic tissue layer clearly distinct from the tendon under

J.A. Nunley (ed.), *The Achilles Tendon: Treatment and Rehabilitation*,
DOI: 10.1007/978-1-387-79206-4_2, © Springer Science + Business Media, LLC 2009

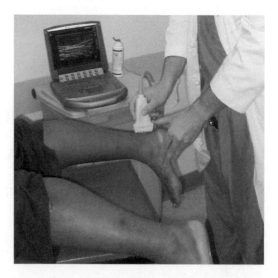

Fig. 2.1. Recommended patient positioning for Achilles ultrasound examination

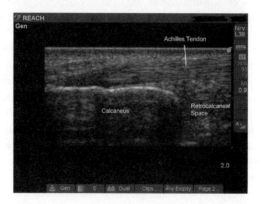

Fig. 2.2. Longitudinal imaging of a normal Achilles tendon insertion

dynamic imaging. The sural nerve and accompanying lesser saphenous vein course from medial to lateral and proximally to distally along the tendon. The plantaris tendon runs along the medial side of the tendon distally. Deep to the Achilles tendon lies the bipennate muscle belly of the flexor hallucis longus.

In most cases, a diagnosis can be made based on the two-dimensional (2D) real-time appearance of the tendon; an acutely ruptured Achilles tendon is clearly identified by a discontinuity of collagen fibrils separated by hypoechoic hematoma (Fig. 2.3). Chronic ruptures demonstrate attenuation of the tendon and echogenic fat herniating into the defect (Fig. 2.4). The calcification and tendinosis pathognomonic of insertional disease can be easily correlated with physical examination findings (Fig. 2.5). In insertional disease, the examiner may use the transducer to palpate and image the osseotendinous junction simultaneously. It should be stressed that all findings must be confirmed in two planes.

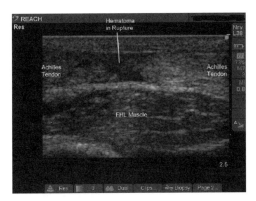

Fig. 2.3. Longitudinal imaging of an acute (24-hour) complete Achilles tendon rupture. FHL, flexor hallucis longus

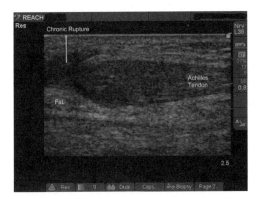

Fig. 2.4. Longitudinal imaging of a chronic (3-month) complete Achilles tendon rupture

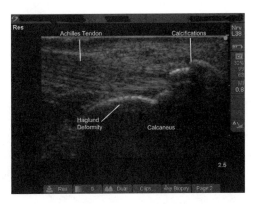

Fig. 2.5. Insertional Achilles tendinosis. Note the tendinopathic enlargement of the Achilles tendon, the prominent Haglund deformity, and insertional calcifications

Additional Diagnostic Techniques

Additional techniques can enhance the diagnosis of Achilles tendon pathology.

Absolute Tendon Size

Some studies have suggested that measurements of tendon thickness may correlate with tendinopathy.[1] Tendon thickness measurements should be obtained directly in the transverse plane. It is generally agreed that the Achilles tendon should not exceed 6 mm in the anteroposterior dimension.[2,3] The diagnosis of Achilles tendinosis can be made in those tendons measuring thicker than 6 mm (Fig. 2.6).

Color/Power Doppler

Color/power Doppler imaging can theoretically demonstrate hyperemia, increased vascularity, and varicosities. The ability to detect blood cell motion also allows the examiner to quickly distinguish if a hypoechoic structure is a vessel or a fluid-filled cyst. Several studies have examined the use of Doppler imaging in the assessment of "tendonitis."[2,4] Although threshold values have been proposed, we have found that an examination of the normal contralateral tendon yields the best comparison for the diagnosis of tendonitis. In this comparison technique, the Doppler signal gain is dialed down at the same location on the contralateral tendon. Reexamination of the symptomatic side while keeping the same gain setting allows the presence of increased blood flow to be easily identified (Fig. 2.7). Although Achilles tendinopathy is usually of the noninflammatory tendinosis type, we have found color Doppler examination useful in the determination of patient compliance with local nitrous oxide treatment for nodular disease.[4–8]

Surrounding Structures

Ultrasound affords excellent visualization of the retrocalcaneal bursa. Because the retrocalcaneal bursa normally contains minimal fluid, a longitudinal image of the Achilles tendon insertion at the calcaneus should demonstrate hyperechoic fat only in the retrocalcaneal bursa. An older study has suggested that distention of the bursa with greater than 3 mm of hypoechoic fluid in any plane is abnormal and consistent with bursitis.[9] In our experience, the clinical correlation of pain with transducer-applied palpation along with the finding of increased fluid (hypoechoic) in the retrocalcaneal area (Fig. 2.8) correlates

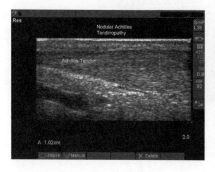
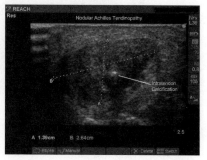

A   B

Fig. 2.6. Longitudinal (A) and transverse (B) imaging of nodular Achilles tendinopathy. Note the fusiform enlargement of the diseased tendon (1.02 cm; and 2.64 cm × 1.39 cm, respectively)

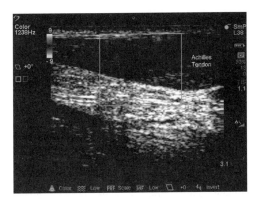

Fig. 2.7. Color Doppler image of Achilles tendinosis treated for 3 months with transdermal nitrous oxide. Note the increased blood flow in the peritendinous tissue. Tendinitis would be similar in appearance

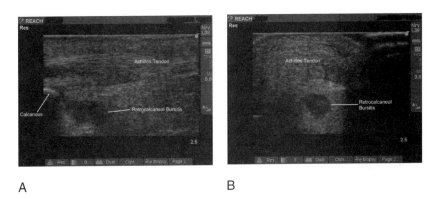

A   B

Fig. 2.8. Longitudinal (A) and transverse (B) imaging of retrocalcaneal bursitis

well with the diagnosis and guided injection of retrocalcaneal bursitis.[10] The use of color/power Doppler imaging may also show hypervascularity in the setting of bursitis.

Diagnosis and Treatment of Achilles Tendinopathy

Fusiform thickening of the Achilles tendon, lakes of hypoechoic tissue, and disruption of the hyperechoic fibrillar ultrastructure are diagnostic of Achilles tendinopathy (tendinosis, tendonitis). Ultrasound images can also be used to help map skin areas for the placement of transdermal nitroderm patches as well as to define, both peri- and intraoperatively, abnormal areas during the surgical debridement of tendinopathic tissue.

Ruptures

Tears in the Achilles tendon manifest as discrete anechoic areas between normal hyperechoic tendon fibers. On transverse imaging, a partial tear involves only a portion of the cross-sectional area of the tendon, while a full tear demonstrates complete discontinuity (Figs. 2.3 and 2.4). Dynamic imaging of the defect during active or passive dorsiplantar flexion can provide a real-time Thompson test, in which the tendon gap widens and narrows. Fractures of

Table 2.1. Risks and benefits of ultrasound[10,12].

Benefits
- Painless and noninvasive
- Inexpensive and relatively easy to use
- Does not use ionizing radiation
- Provides real-time imaging, making it an excellent surgical tool for guiding minimally invasive procedures, such as cortisone injections, needle biopsies, and aspiration of fluid in joints or elsewhere
- Not affected by cardiac pacemakers, ferromagnetic implants, or metallic fragments within the body
- Small probe and machine footprint yield an excellent alternative to magnetic resonance imaging (MRI) for claustrophobic patients
- Advantages over MRI in seeing tendon structure; some studies have suggested that ultrasound better appreciates tendon structure than MRI[10]
- Can be performed by orthopedic surgeons at the time of examination, thereby truly localizing the pathology

Risks
- For standard diagnostic ultrasound, there are no known harmful effects
- Need to keep sterile techniques intact in setting of nonsterile ultrasound gel during procedures

the calcaneus can also be visualized in the appropriate individual. It should be noted that ultrasound is particularly good at visualizing fractures around a growth plate and the apophysis in the pediatric population. A prior study has examined the usefulness of ultrasound as a selection tool for judging when or when not to proceed with surgical versus conservative treatment for acute Achilles tendon ruptures.[11] Dynamic ultrasound may allow for better judgment on which patients would benefit from surgical versus conservative treatment.

Guided Procedures

Minimally invasive percutaneous ultrasound-guided interventions may be performed both in the office and operative settings. As with any new surgical technique, we recommend practice in the cadaveric lab to gain familiarity and facility. The presence of ultrasound gel leads to some potential hazards for our patients. Sterility should be maintained at all times. Depending on the procedure, we have found the use of sterile transducer covers and sterile coupling gel to be effective in maintaining a sterile field. With careful technique, nonsterile gel and transducer can be sequestered from the sterile field.

Troubleshooting

Tendons are anisotropic (they look different depending on the direction in which the ultrasound beam is angled). If the transducer is not properly aligned perpendicular to the tendon, a falsely hypoechoic image of the tendon will be obtained, mimicking tendinopathy (Table 2.1).

References

1. Richards PJ, Dheerak, McCall IM. Achilles tendon size and power Doppler ultrasound changes compared to MRI: a preliminary observational study. Clin Radiol 2001;56(10):843–50.
2. Richards PJ, Win T, Jones PW. The distribution of microvascular response in Achilles tendonopathy assessed by colour and power Doppler. Skeletal Radiol 2005;34(6):336–42.

3. Bjordal JM, Lopes-Martins RA, Iversen VV. A randomised, placebo controlled trial of low level laser therapy for activated Achilles tendinitis with microdialysis measurement of peritendinous prostaglandin E2 concentrations. Br J Sports Med 2006;40(1):76–80.
4. Knobloch K, Kraemer R, Lichtenberg A, et al. Achilles tendon and paratendon microcirculation in midportion and insertional tendinopathy in athletes. Am J Sports Med 2006;34(1):92–7.
5. Paoloni JA, Appleyard RC, Nelson J, et al. Topical glyceryl trinitrate treatment of chronic noninsertional Achilles tendinopathy. A randomized, double-blind, placebo-controlled trial. J Bone Joint Surg Am 2004;86A(5):916–22.
6. Ozgocmen S, Kiris A, Ardicoglu O, et al. Glucocorticoid iontophoresis for Achilles tendon enthesitis in ankylosing spondylitis: significant response documented by power Doppler ultrasound. Rheumatol Int 2005;25(2):158–60.
7. Murrell GA, Szabo C, Hannafin JA, et al. Modulation of tendon healing by nitric oxide. Inflamm Res 1997;46(1):19–27.
8. Hunte G, Lloyd-Smith R. Topical glyceryl trinitrate for chronic Achilles tendinopathy. Clin J Sports Med 2005;15(2):116–7.
9. Ozgocmen S, Kiris A, Kocakoc E, et al. Evaluation of metacarpophalangeal joint synovitis in rheumatoid arthritis by power Doppler technique: relationship between synovial vascularization and periarticular bone mineral density. Joint Bone Spine 2004;71(5):384–8.
10. Nazarian LN, Rawool NM, Martin CE, et al. Synovial fluid in the hindfoot and ankle: detection of amount and distribution with US. Radiology 1995;197(1):275–8.
11. Jacobson JA. Musculoskeletal ultrasound and MRI: which do I choose? Semin Musculoskelet Radiol 2005;9(2):135–49.
12. RadiologyInfo. Radiological Society of North America, Inc. (RSNA), 2007 http://www.radiologyinfo.org/en/info.cfm?pg=musculous8bhcp=1.

3

Magnetic Resonance Imaging of the Achilles Tendon

Kush Singh and Clyde A. Helms

Clinical Indications

Several different clinical scenarios warrant evaluation of the Achilles tendon with magnetic resonance imaging (MRI). However, the main reasons to image the Achilles are pain, trauma, infection, or a mass. Less commonly, an MRI may be used to screen for hypercholesterolemia. Although a diagnosis of Achilles tendon rupture is usually evident clinically, the gap between the ruptured ends of the tendon may be difficult to ascertain by physical examination alone. This gap is frequently used to determine which technique will be employed for surgical repair. When the gap is small, and the injury acute, then nonoperative management may be selected (see Chapter 5). In the chronic rupture, when the gap is less than 6 cm, the augmentation techniques can be applied and when the gap is greater than 6 cm, then tendon transfer is selected. It is often useful for the surgeon to know which technique will be best utilized for preoperative planning, and in these situations MRI can be quite helpful.

Technique

When imaging the ankle using MRI, the standard ankle protocol should be used. Slight variations in the ankle protocol are used to optimize visualization of the Achilles tendon, including a wider field of view, which should include the musculotendinous junction of the Achilles tendon. Standard technique includes a combination of T1-weighted (T1W) and some type of T2-weighted (T2W) sequence in all three orthogonal planes. Typically, a fast spine echo (FSE) T2W image with fat saturation is used for the T2W sequence. Contrast is rarely, if ever, used unless there is suspected infection or concern of a mass (to differentiate solid from cystic).

Normal Tendon

The normal Achilles tendon demonstrates low signal intensity on all pulse sequences. Commonly, there is a solitary vertical line of high signal intensity

J.A. Nunley (ed.), *The Achilles Tendon: Treatment and Rehabilitation*,
DOI: 10.1007/978-1-387-79206-4_3, © Springer Science+Business Media, LLC 2009

in the midsubstance of the tendon, which probably represents the site where the soleus and gastrocnemius tendons are apposed to one another, or else it represents a vascular channel.

Artifacts

Increased signal may be seen within the tendon in pathologic conditions as well as with artifacts. Two of the most common artifacts seen when imaging the Achilles tendon are insertional signal and the magic angle phenomenon.

Insertional signal is a slightly increased signal intensity near the osseous insertion on the calcaneus from interposed fatty material between the tendon fibers. The magic angle phenomenon is common in MRI and occurs when those tendon fibers oriented at an angle of about 55 degrees to the bore of the magnet demonstrate high signal intensity on short echo time (TE) sequences.[1] Short TE sequences include T1W, proton density, and gradient echo (GRE) sequences. This artifact may be distinguished from pathology by using a pulse sequence with a long TE (causing the intratendinous high signal to disappear), by observing that the tendon is of normal caliber, or by repositioning the lower extremity so that the Achilles tendon is imaged at a different angle relative to the bore of the magnet.

Achilles Pathology

Achilles pathology commonly occurs about 4 cm above the calcaneal insertion, but may exist anywhere along the length of the muscle tendon unit. Tears and degeneration may also occur at the musculotendinous junction (proximal), and the field of view must be large enough to include this region on sagittal images to look for hemorrhage and edema in the acute state, or muscle atrophy in the chronic setting. When tears and degeneration occur at the insertion site of the Achilles tendon (distal), it is called insertional tendinosis/tendinopathy.

Myxoid degeneration occurs from aging or chronic use and is also referred to as tendinosis or tendinopathy. Although it represents a painless process, myxoid degeneration weakens the tendon so that it is predisposed to tears from minimal trauma. On MRI, a degenerated Achilles tendon demonstrates high signal intensity within the substance of the tendon on both T1W and any type of T2W sequence (Fig. 3.1 and Fig. 3.2) Typically, the term *degeneration* (or *tendinosis* or *tendinopathy*) is used when the T2 signal within the substance of the Achilles tendon is not as bright as fluid. When the T2 signal within the substance of the Achilles tendon is brighter than fluid, the term *partial tear* is used.

Paratenonitis and *peritendonitis* are synonymous terms used to describe an inflammatory process in a tendon without a tendon sheath. Magnetic resonance demonstrates abnormal signal intensity typical of edema (low T1, high T2) in the soft tissues surrounding the tendon. This process is similar to tenosynovitis, which is an inflammatory process of a tendon sheath.

Partial Achilles tendon tears represent incomplete disruption of the tendon fibers. When the T2 signal within the substance of the Achilles tendon is brighter than fluid, the term *partial tear* is used (Fig. 3.3). The tendon may be thickened (hypertrophic), thinned (atrophic), or of normal caliber. In a normal-caliber tendon, an abnormal signal may be the only evidence of the partial tear.

An attenuated tendon is closer to complete rupture than a thickened tendon. Tendons frequently become partially torn in a longitudinal or vertical manner, rather than transversely, resulting in a split tendon that may be functionally incompetent (acts as if it is completely torn) even though it is still in continuity with the muscle and the bone. Usually, there is high signal intensity in the tendon on all pulse sequences with partial tears, but with chronic partial tears there may be low signal intensity because of scarring and fibrosis.

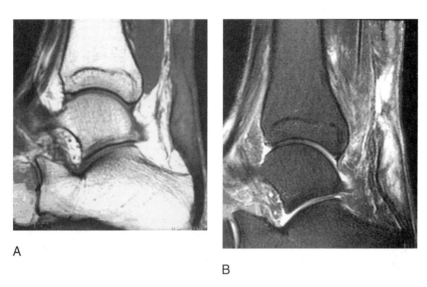

A

B

Fig. 3.1. Sagittal T1-weighted (A) and fast spine echo (FSE) T2-weighted (B) images with fat saturation demonstrate T1 and T2 signal abnormality within the distal Achilles tendon. There is thickening of the tendon without discontinuity of the tendon fibers to suggest a tear. Findings are most consistent with Achilles tendinopathy or tendinosis

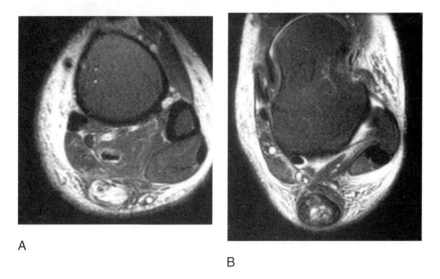

A

B

Fig. 3.2. (A,B) Two separate axial FSE T2-weighted images with fat saturation as well as coronal T1-weighted

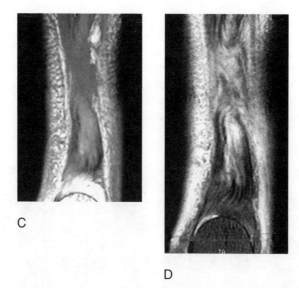

Fig. 3.2. (continued) (C) coronal FSE T2-weighted (D) images. These images again demonstrate T1 and T2 signal abnormality with tendon thickening, most consistent with Achilles tendinopathy or tendinosis

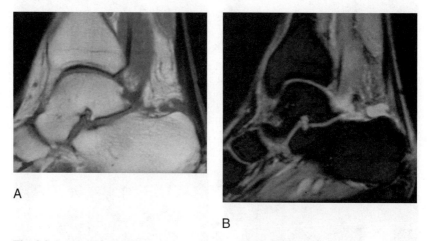

Fig. 3.3. Sagittal T1-weighted (A) and FSE T2-weighted (B) images with fat saturation demonstrate signal abnormality and discontinuity of the anterior fibers of the distal Achilles tendon, consistent with a partial tear of the Achilles tendon. Incidental note is made of retrocalcaneal bursitis

Complete (or full-thickness) tears indicate total disruption of the fibers of the tendon so that there are two separate fragments. Increased T2 signal (brighter than fluid) is also seen, as is additional total disruption of the tendon fibers (Fig. 3.4) It is important to assess both the quality of the remnant tendons and the length of tendon retraction when evaluating complete tendon tears.

Complete tears are usually easy to evaluate and diagnose clinically. However, there is value in imaging these patients in order to evaluate how close the tendon fragments are to one another and to evaluate the condition of

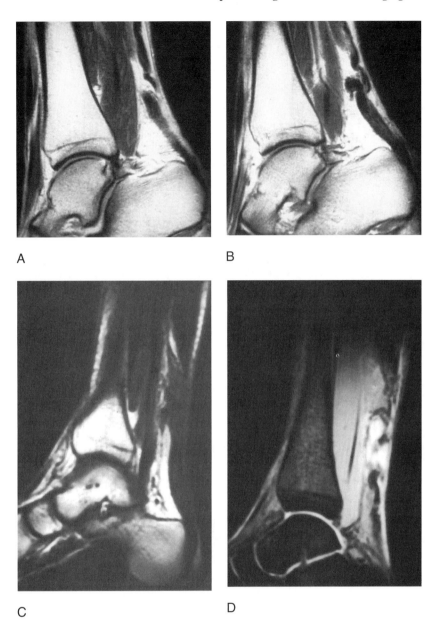

A

B

C

D

Fig. 3.4. (continued)

the tendon. Imaging may be done in a cast, which serves to hold the ankle in plantar flexion, causing increased apposition of tendon fragments.

Two separate bursa are recognized about the Achilles tendon. The retro-calcaneal bursa is a teardrop-shaped structure normally located between the tendon and the posterior aspect of the upper calcaneus (Fig. 3.5) This structure usually contains little or no fluid within it when not inflamed. The tendo-Achilles (retro-Achilles) bursa is an acquired or adventitious bursa, located in the subcutaneous fat dorsal to the Achilles tendon. Haglund's deformity (also known as "pump bumps") consists of a triad of retro-Achilles bursitis, retro-calcaneal bursitis, and thickening of the distal Achilles tendon. This condition

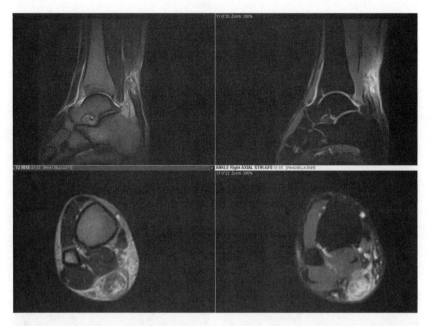

E

Fig. 3.4. (continued) (A,B) Sagittal T1-weighted images of the ankle demonstrate complete disruption of the fibers of the distal Achilles tendon with associated laxity, consistent with a complete tear. (C) Sagittal T1 and FSE T2-weighted image also demonstrate complete disruption of the fibers of the distal Achilles tendon with associated laxity, consistent with a complete tear. Sagittal (D) and axial (E) FSE T2-weighted images with fat saturation as well as short tau inversion recovery (STIR), a type of T2-weighting (F), image again demonstrate findings of a complete Achilles tendon tear

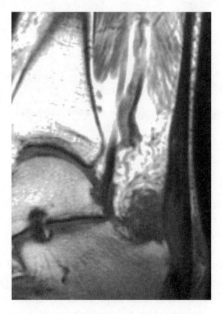

Fig. 3.5. Sagittal T1-weighted image demonstrates low T1 signal, rounded structure posterior to the calcaneus and anterior to the Achilles tendon (arrow), most consistent with retrocalcaneal bursitis

is commonly seen in the setting of chronic overuse, especially from ill-fitting footwear, hence the term *pump bumps*.[2]

With any inflammatory condition of the heel, especially when symptoms occur bilaterally, one must always consider systemic inflammatory disease as a possible etiology. Such symptoms are not uncommonly seen with rheumatoid arthritis, ankylosing spondylitis, and Reiter's syndrome, among others. In fact, retrocalcaneal bursitis has been noted to occur in up to 10% of patients who have rheumatoid arthritis.[34]

Xanthomas occur in the setting of familial hyperlipidemia types II and III (hypercholesterolemia and hypertriglyceridemia). Xanthomas result when intermediate signal intensity lipid-laden foamy histiocytes infiltrate between low signal intensity tendon fibers (Fig. 3.6) They have a predilection for the Achilles tendon as well as the extensor tendons of the hand. Imaging characteristics are very similar to partial tendon tears, including diffuse thickening and high signal on T1W and T2W images with a stippled appearance representing infiltrating fat. Distinguishing features of a xanthoma include bilaterality and abnormal laboratory values indicating elevated cholesterol levels. Often, the two processes are indistinguishable.[5]

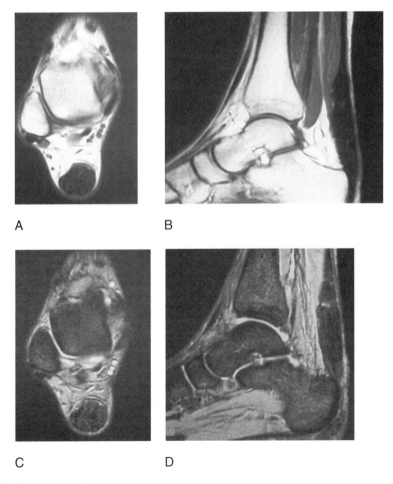

A

B

C

D

Fig. 3.6. (continued)

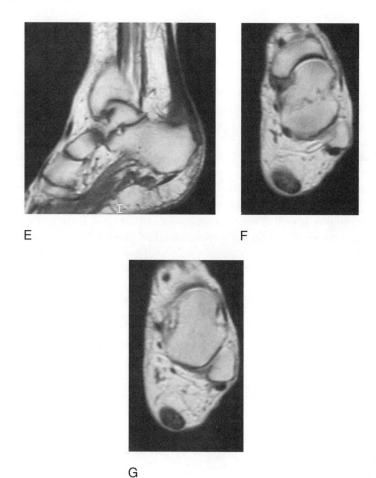

Fig. 3.6. Axial (A) and sagittal (B) T1-weighted and FSE T2-weighted images (C,D) demonstrate thickening and signal abnormality within the distal Achilles tendon. Findings could be related to partial tendon tears or xanthomas. These were xanthomas in this patient with familial hyperlipidemia. Sagittal (E) and axial (F,G) T1-weighted images also demonstrate the speckled and thickened appearance of a xanthoma within the Achilles tendon. These findings could easily be confused with a partial tendon tear without the appropriate clinical history

References

1. Chandnani VP, Bradley YC. Achilles tendon and miscellaneous tendon lesions. Magn Reson Imaging Clin North Am 1994;2(1):89–96.
2. Pavlov H, Heneghan MA, Hersh A, et al. The Haglund syndrome: initial and differential diagnosis. Radiology 1982;144(1):83–8.
3. Gerster JC, Vischer TL, Bennani A, et al. The painful heel. Comparative study in rheumatoid arthritis, ankylosing spondylitis, Reiter's syndrome, and generalized osteoarthrosis. Ann Rheum Dis 1977;36(4):343–8.
4. Turlik MA. Seronegative arthritis as a cause of heel pain. Clin Podiatr Med Surg 1990;7(2):369–75.
5. Dussault RG, Kaplan PA, Roederer G. MR imaging of Achilles tendon in patients with familial hyperlipidemia: comparison with plain films, physical examination, and patients with traumatic tendon lesions. AJR Am J Roentgenol 1995;164(2):403–7.

Section II

Acute Injuries

4

Ruptures of the Medial Gastrocnemius Muscle ("Tennis Leg")

Joseph Yu and William E. Garrett, Jr.

In 1883, Powell[1] first reported in *The Lancet* on the "lawn tennis leg" (rupture of the medial head of the gastrocnemius). He described a 41-year-old healthy man who had sudden, sharp pain when reaching for the ball while playing tennis. Pain, tenderness, and swelling rapidly developed, but the patient was able to return to sports in 4 weeks. In 1958, Arner and Lindholm[2] surgically explored five of 20 patients with tennis leg. In each case, a transverse rupture of the medial gastrocnemius at the musculotendinous junction was found.

Ruptures of the medial head of the gastrocnemius muscle have been documented in patients ranging from adolescents to the elderly. The incidence is greatest in the middle-aged, as reported by Millar,[3] who reported a mean age of 42 years for men and 46 for women, which suggests a degenerative process analogous to a rupture of the long head of the biceps, the rotator cuff of the shoulder, the Achilles tendon, or the attachment of the rectus femoris.[4] Ruptures to the medial head of the gastrocnemius are nearly nonexistent in young tennis players with the same stresses.[5] This injury seems to be most common in men.

The term *tennis leg* arose because many patients suffering this injury were playing tennis at the time of injury. To understand why tennis leg is an injury of the middle-aged tennis player, one needs to consider the factors that may cause the gastrocnemius muscle to stretch and rupture. The flat-heeled tennis shoe allows excessive ankle dorsiflexion, which tightens the heel cord distally, while sudden knee extension increases the tension on the muscle belly proximally.[6] Tennis is an active cutting sport that requires players to perform sudden movements that place the gastrocnemius in a position of risk. Of sports in which this age group generally participates, golf, swimming, walking, and jogging are not cutting sports. Other sports that do require cutting, such as football, basketball, and soccer, usually do not have much participation by individuals in their 40s and 50s in the United States.

J.A. Nunley (ed.), *The Achilles Tendon: Treatment and Rehabilitation*,
DOI: 10.1007/978-1-387-79206-4_4, © Springer Science+Business Media, LLC 2009

Anatomy

Muscles such as the gastrocnemius, the biceps femoris, and the rectus femoris are quite vulnerable to injury because they cross two joints and are subjected to excessive stretch.[7] Ruptures of the medial gastrocnemius occur where the medial head of the gastrocnemius inserts into the soleus aponeurosis (Fig. 4.1). In the position of knee extension and ankle dorsiflexion, the gastrocnemius muscle is stretched to its maximum length, increasing the tension on the muscle.[6] A powerful contraction of the gastrocnemius muscle with concomitant overstretching of the muscle leads to excessive tensile force and disruption of the musculotendinous junction.[8]

Muscle injury due to indirect or strain injury occurs near the junction of the muscle fibers to the tendon. A normal tendon does not tear in response to excess strain. The tear occurs within the muscle fibers close to the tendon. Stretch is needed to create injury; muscle activation alone is insufficient to create macro-injury.[8]

Clinical Presentation

The classic description of a ruptured gastrocnemius includes a sudden contraction of the muscle with the ankle dorsiflexed and the knee extended. The patient is commonly a middle-aged man who complains of acute, sports-related pain in

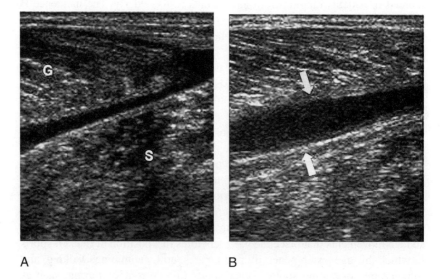

A   B

Fig. 4.1. A complete rupture of the medial head of the gastrocnemius. (A) The longitudinal ultrasound image obtained 1 day after the injury is characterized by blunting of the triangular taper of the gastrocnemius tendon (G) to its insertion onto the soleus muscle (S). This is accompanied by disruption of the normal parallel linear echogenic and hypoechogenic lines within the tendon insertion. (B) An ultrasound image obtained 4 weeks later shows the union of the hypoechoic tissue between the distal ends of the medial head of the gastrocnemius with the soleus muscle (arrows). (From Kwak HS. Diagnosis and follow-up US evaluation of ruptures of the medial head of the gastrocnemius ("tennis leg"). Korean J Radiol 2006;7:193–8, with permission.)

the middle portion of the calf. It is not unusual for a patient to say that it felt as if he had been hit in the calf by an errant ball from an adjacent tennis court. The injury has also been documented after minimal trauma, such as stepping off a curb,[4] where the patient complains of an acute episode of sharp pain in the calf. A prodrome of calf pain a day or two before the injury may exist.[6,11] Froimson[6] questioned his patients specifically about this, and nearly half recalled prodromic calf discomfort. Pain is increased with attempted jumping, sudden passive ankle dorsiflexion, or active plantarflexion of the ankle.

Examination reveals maximal tenderness over the musculotendinous junction of the medial gastrocnemius. Usually, a sulcus or depression is observed at the site of rupture. Fifty years ago, Arner and Lindholm[2] reported 20 cases of rupture of the medial head of the gastrocnemius at the musculotendinous insertion; in each case it was possible to feel a defect at the midcalf. Swelling can be variable and may obscure the defect. Within a few days, ecchymosis may appear in the area as well. However, the ecchymosis may also move distally because of gravity and the dependent foot position. Plantar flexion strength is diminished, and there is decreased muscle tone in the medial head of the gastrocnemius.[6] However, a negative Thompson test is noted.[12,13].

There are two reports of tennis leg leading to acute compartment syndrome.[14,15] In both cases, the patients were middle-aged, and they suffered sports-related injuries. Elevated compartment pressures were obtained in the anterior, lateral, and posterior compartments, but not in the deep posterior compartment. During the fasciotomy, Jarolem et al.[13] found a tear in the medial gastrocnemius musculotendinous junction and a large, secondary hematoma. The cases demonstrate that compartment syndrome has been reported as a result of tennis leg, and the treating physician should be aware of that. However, the fascia overlying the medial gastrocnemius is relatively thin, and there is some question regarding the likelihood of sustaining pressures in the superficial compartment that are capable of causing ischemic muscle injury.

Case Study

A 38-year-old man was playing doubles tennis when a short shot was returned to him. As he transitioned from moving side-to-side to suddenly moving forward, he felt a sharp sensation in his midcalf posteriorly. He looked for a ball or a racquet that might have hit him there to explain the sudden pop, but he saw nothing. He noticed increasing pain in the calf. His heel cord felt intact, and he could move his ankle in plantar and dorsiflexion. When he started to walk, he felt a sharp pain near toe-off as his foot dorsiflexed and his knee extended. He could not walk on tiptoe.

His tennis foursome included an orthopedic surgeon who suggested a heel lift and a short course of nonsteroidal antiinflammatory medications. The foursome also included a radiologist who suggested a magnetic resonance imaging (MRI) examination due to concern about a partial Achilles tendon injury. The MRI showed edema and inflammation openly at the musculotendinous junction of the medial head of the gastrocnemius.

The patient later noted ecchymosis in the calf, ankle, and toes after several days. He limped for about 2 weeks and then could walk nearly normally. He started stretching and strengthening. In about 6 weeks he could play tennis cautiously, and at 8 weeks he felt recovered.

Imaging

Not surprisingly, roentgenographic examination of these injuries is normal. With an adequate clinical examination, radiographs should not be necessary, but may be needed to rule out other conditions.

In a normal patient, an ultrasound examination demonstrates the normal taper of the distal medial gastrocnemius muscle superficial to the soleus muscle. A tear of the medial gastrocnemius muscle is characterized by disruption of the normal parallel linear echogenic and hypoechogenic appearance of the tendon. This is accompanied by an indistinct tapering of the tendon's distal end at its insertion.[16] Sometimes a hematoma is seen as hypoechogenic material, with posterior acoustic enhancement seen at the insertion site.

Magnetic resonance images show an abnormality of the medial part of the gastrocnemius. T1-weighted images may show disruption of the normal architecture of the musculotendinous junction while T2-weighted images show increased signal in the injured muscle due to edema (Fig. 4.2). A hematoma can appear as a homogeneous or heterogeneous mass on the image. The hematoma is visible as a high-intensity signal on T1- and T2-weighted scans[17] that can be seen tracking along the epimysium.[18] Magnetic resonance imaging is usually unnecessary, but can be helpful in differentiating between tennis leg and other conditions such as deep vein thrombosis and a partial Achilles tendon rupture.

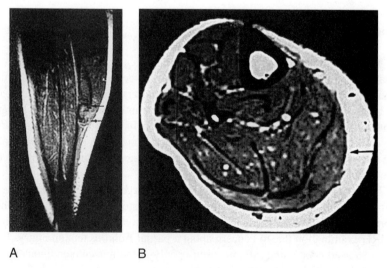

A   B

Fig. 4.2. Magnetic resonance images of the affected leg. (A) T1-weighted coronal section, revealing the hematoma and torn muscle in the medial part of the gastrocnemius (arrows). (B) T1-weighted cross section showing an altered signal in the medial part of the gastrocnemius (arrow). (From Menz and Lucas,[16] with permission.)

Differential Diagnosis

The swelling from a medial gastrocnemius rupture is easily confused with thrombophlebitis or deep vein thrombosis,[4],[19] which demonstrate similar clinical manifestations such as calf swelling, tenderness, and pain with dorsiflexion of the ankle. If there is any question, the easily performed duplex scan is a very accurate method to assess thrombophlebitis. A misdiagnosis may result in unnecessary anticoagulation therapy. Anouchi et al.[18] describes a case report in which a patient with a rupture of the medial head of the gastrocnemius was administered heparin for a presumptive diagnosis of thrombophlebitis. The patient developed a large hematoma and posterior compartment syndrome in his calf. The most common mistake is to neglect the history and jump to a conclusion of thrombophlebitis or deep vein thrombosis. In most cases, a careful history should be enough to reach the correct diagnosis.

The very existence of a plantaris tendon rupture used to be questioned,[20] but recently it has been documented surgically[21] and by MRI.[22],[23] The musculotendinous junction of the plantaris is in the lateral popliteal area that is overlapped by the lateral gastrocnemius and therefore is distant from the medial calf defect.[2] Rupture of this small tendon typically does not lead to the pain, bleeding, and swelling that characterizes a rupture of the gastrocnemius. Further, plantarflexion weakness would not be associated with ruptures of the plantaris.[2] Surgeons who harvest the plantaris tendon for flexor tendon grafting report that patients experience only transitory popliteal tenderness and minimal calf pain without weakness or inability to walk normally.[6]

Treatment

There are no randomized controlled studies comparing nonoperative and operative treatment. Although surgical treatment has been recommended,[2],[3] most surgeons[24],[25] recommend conservative management with these injuries. Without surgery, the prognosis for this injury is excellent and permanent disability is extremely rare. In a series of 720 patients, rehabilitation had only a 0.7% recurrence rate.[3] Shields et al.[10] compared the isokinetic performance of the injured leg with that of the normal leg following conservative treatment and reported no significant loss in plantarflexion strength in the injured extremity after healing.[11]

Applying a heel wedge[6] or an ankle-foot orthosis in slight plantarflexion[24] alleviates discomfort by reducing the strain on the injured gastrocnemius. Also because the heel is elevated, the limb seems a bit longer. This keeps the patient's knee slightly flexed, further relaxing the gastrocnemius muscle belly.[6] Early treatment with ice and antiinflammatory drugs has been reported to decrease recovery time in patients with tennis leg.[3] Kwak et al.[25] applied an early compressive dressing after muscle rupture and found that a neoprene cast sleeve significantly decreased the amount of hematoma fluid collection, allowing earlier ambulation. Patients in the compressive group also developed a union between the medial head of the gastrocnemius with the soleus muscle more rapidly, as verified by ultrasonography (4.25 versus 3.25 weeks; $p <.05$).

Rest is recommended during the acute inflammatory phase (1 to 5 days after injury).[18] Beginning a few days after the injury, with the knee fully extended, the posterior calf musculature can be passively stretched to tolerance with a towel. Isometric ankle dorsiflexion and plantarflexion can also begin at this time. Passive stretching can be replaced with a standing stretch of the ankle at 2 weeks. Resistive strengthening exercises against a rubberband are also begun. Most clinicians report resumption of athletic activities at 4 to 6 weeks. Patients should be cautioned that full recovery could take up to 16 weeks.

References

1. Powell RM. . Lawn tennis leg. Lancet 1883;2:44.
2. Arner O, Lindholm A. What is tennis leg? Acta Chir Scand 1958;116:73–7.
3. Millar AP. Strains of the posterior calf musculature ("tennis leg"). Am J Sports Med 1979;7:172–4.
4. McClure JG. Gastrocnemius musculotendinous rupture: a condition confused with thrombophlebitis. South Med J 77(9):1143–5.
5. Hutchinson MR, Laprade RF, Burnett QM. Injury surveillance at the USTA boys' tennis championships: a 6-year study. Med Sci Sports Exerc 1995;7:826–30.
6. Froimson AI. Tennis leg. JAMA 1969;209:415–6.
7. Brewer BJ. Mechanism of injury to the musculotendinous unit. In: Instructional Course Lectures, vol 17. St. Louis: CV Mosby, 354–8.
8. Nikolaou PK, Macdonald BL, Glisson RR, et al. Biomechanical and histological evaluation of muscle after controlled strain injury. Am J Sports Med 1987;15:9–14.
9. Gilbert TJ Jr, Bullis BR, Griffiths HJ. Tennis calf or tennis leg. Orthopedics 1996;19:179–84.
10. Shields CL, Redix L, Brester CE. Acute tears of the medial head of the gastrocnemius. Foot Ankle 1985;5:186–90.
11. Thompson TC, Doherty JH. Spontaneous rupture of the tendon of Achilles: a new clinical diagnostic test. J Trauma 1962;2:126–9.
12. Durig M, Schuppisser, Schuppisser JP, et al. Spontaneous rupture of the gastrocnemius muscle. Injury 1997;9:143–5.
13. Jarolem KL, Wolinsky PR, Savenor A, et al. Tennis leg leading to acute compartment syndrome. Orthopedics 1994;17:721–3.
14. Straehley D, Jones W. Acute compartment syndrome (anterior, lateral, and superficial posterior) following tear of the medial head of the gastrocnemius muscle. A case report. Am J Sports Med 1986;14:96–9.
15. Jamadar DA, Jacobson JA, Theisen SE, et al. Sonography of the painful calf: differential considerations. Am J Roentgenol 2002;179:709–16.
16. Menz MJ, Lucas GL. Magnetic resonance imaging of a rupture of the medial head of the gastrocnemius muscle. A case report. J Bone Joint Surg [Am] 1991;73:1260–2.
17. Noonan TJ, Garrett WE Jr. Muscle strain injury: diagnosis and treatment. J Am Acad Orthop Surg 1999;7:262–9.
18. Anouchi YS, Parker RD, Seitz WH. Posterior compartment syndrome of the calf resulting from misdiagnosis of a rupture of the medial head of the gastrocnemius. J Trauma 1987;27:678–80.
19. Severance HW Jr, Bassett FH 3rd. Rupture of the plantaris—does it exist? J Bone Joint Surg [Am] 1982;64:1387–8.
20. Hamilton W, Klostermeier T, Lim EV, et al. Surgically documented rupture of the plantaris muscle: a case report and literature review. Foot Ankle Int 1997;18:522–3.
21. Helms CA, Fritz RC, Garvin GJ. Plantaris muscle injury: evaluation with MR imaging. Musculoskel Radiol 1995;195:201–3.
22. Allard JC, Bancroft J, Porter G. Imaging of plantaris muscle ruptures. Clin Imaging 1992;16:55–8.
23. Johnson EW. Tennis leg. Am J Phys Med Rehabil 2000;79:221.
24. Leach RE. Leg and foot injuries in racquet sports. Clin Sports Med 1988;7:359–70.
25. Kwak HS, Lee KB, Han YM. Ruptures of the medial head of the gastrocnemius ("tennis leg"): clinical outcome and compression effect. Clin Imaging 2006;30:48–53.

5

Nonoperative Management of Acute Ruptures

Hajo Thermann and Christoph Becher

The rapidly growing trend for participation in recreational and competitive sports is accompanied by an increase of overuse syndromes. In the foot and ankle, the incidence of Achilles tendon ruptures and tendon-related disorders has increased significantly in the last decades.[1–3] In Germany alone, the incidence of acute Achilles tendon rupture is estimated to be 15,000 cases a year.[3]

The classic Achilles rupture usually does not occur at times of the highest level of sports activities, but rather shows a peak incidence between the ages of 30 and 45 years.[4–9] This patient population is made up of a remarkably large portion of leisure athletes and patients with sedentary occupations.[10] In the athletic population, the portion of injuries among track-and-field athletes is cited as only 10%, and these are mostly young patients who have sustained a tendon rupture as a result of an incompletely treated Achilles tendinopathy or after an enormous training workload.[9]

In the future, an increasing number of older patients (over 50 years) will sustain acute Achilles tendon ruptures, as strenuous sports activities become more and more normal in this age group, and since the Achilles tendon seems to be one of the tendons that is most susceptible to degenerative changes within the human body. The male-to-female ratio of Achilles tendon ruptures ranges between 5:1 and 10:1 in most series, and, on average, the men are older than the women.[9,11]

According to the literature and the authors' experience, an Achilles tendon rupture most frequently (80% to 90% of cases) occurs 2 to 6 cm proximal to its calcaneal insertion.[9] The incidence of proximal ruptures at the musculotendinous junction is 10% to 15%, and the ruptures are usually caused by degenerative changes. Ruptures at or near the calcaneal insertion are rare and are mostly found in patients who are hyperpronators and who have a large Haglund's deformity or in individuals who have received a steroid injection for the treatment of tendinopathy. Most typical intratendinous ruptures occur because of a rapid loading of the tendon, but bony avulsions are caused by continuously increasing tension and strength on the heel or by direct impact.[9] The classic rupture mechanism is usually a consequence of an indirect loading and traction mechanism such as during push-off with the foot in plantarflexion with simultaneous knee extension, or with a sudden, unexpected dorsiflexion of the

J.A. Nunley (ed.), *The Achilles Tendon: Treatment and Rehabilitation*,
DOI: 10.1007/978-1-387-79206-4_5, © Springer Science+Business Media, LLC 2009

ankle with powerful contraction of the calf muscles.[9] Direct impact, such as a kick or hit on the tensed tendon, accounts for only 1% to 10% of ruptures.[11,12] The degenerative and the mechanical theories of the pathogenesis of Achilles tendon rupture are continually debated. Aseptic inflammations (tendinitis, paratendinosis) and reduced vascular supply lead to degenerative changes with cell loss and disorders of mucopolysaccharide content, even progressing to fatty, mucoid, or calcifying degeneration of the tendon.[13] Repetitive or single stresses result in minor microtrauma. Low temperature and fatigue of athletes leads to a decreased maximal load resistance of the tendon, causing injury.[9] If the regenerative healing processes cannot keep pace with injury, the sum of microtrauma leads to rupture.

Diagnosis

Typical patients with an acute tendon rupture feel as though they have been struck in the calf with an object. The pain is quite intense. Ruptures happening in contact sports often feel as though the player has been struck by a bat or ball on the back of the calf. A crack or a popping sound is often heard or perceived by the player. On physical examination, a palpable gap in the tendon and a positive Thompson test are the first clinical signs of an acute Achilles tendon rupture. Because of hematoma formation, these signs are not always visible but usually are palpable. The patient should be examined in the prone position to facilitate the diagnosis. The strength of ankle plantarflexion is typically decreased or completely lost with an acute rupture, which results in an inability to perform a heel rise and there is weak rolling of the foot with walking. Frequently, the foot is externally rotated as well. Retraining plantarflexion strength at the ankle does not indicate an intact Achilles tendon since the extrinsic flexors, such as the flexor digitorum longus and flexor hallucis longus, are also able to produce this movement.

Although most Achilles tendon ruptures can be diagnosed clinically, evaluation by ultrasonography and magnetic resonance imaging (MRI) enables a definitive diagnosis and can be helpful for the selection of treatment. The ultrasonographic appearance of acute Achilles tendon rupture shows broad variations. The most common signs are interruption of continuity and well-demarcated tendon stumps. Hypoechogenic accumulations of liquid at the rupture site and loss of the typical parallel hyperechogenic reflex patterns are seen regularly by experienced examiners. As some ruptures do not show a visible diastasis of the tendon stumps from the hematoma, dynamic examination in dorsiflexion and plantarflexion is essential (Figs. 5.1A, B). Even if there is no visible gap of the injured tendon, a spreading of fine parallel echoes, corresponding to a loss of the crosswise network of elastic fibers, reveals a rupture. Inflammatory tendinosis with edematous dissolution of these structures has to be differentiated from acute ruptures. Disrupted or retracted soleus fibers, which are detected mostly in high-level athletes, are significant for the choice of treatment and especially for surgical management. Although Achilles rupture can be detected and seen by ultrasonography, MRI allows for the best visualization.[9] The soleus muscle has to be examined with sagittal and axial scans. Furthermore, the differentiation of the rupture area and tendon ends enables an exact determination of the diastasis of the tendon ends and the distance to the calcaneal insertion.

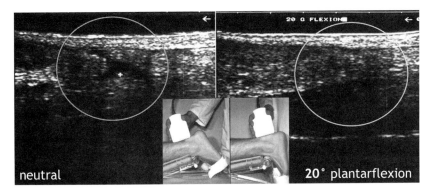

A

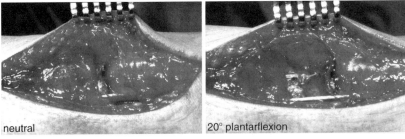

B

Fig. 5.1. (A) Gapping in 0 degrees and complete tendon adaptation at 20 degrees of plantarflexion. (B) Gapping in 0 degrees and complete tendon adaptation at 20c degrees of plantarflexion in situ

The final test, which proves nonfunctioning of the Achilles/soleus/gastrocnemius complex, is the inability to perform a single heel rise, even when radiologic diagnosis (by MRI or ultrasonography) describes a partial rupture.

Treatment

Primary nonoperative immobilization treatment with prolonged care in a cast is no longer justified because of the disadvantages of muscle atrophy and loss of coordination, proprioception, and joint stiffness that must occur with cast treatment. Our concept of primary functional treatment relies on the ultrasound or MRI morphology as an obligatory basis for our treatment strategy to be treated nonoperatively, as follows:

1. The ultrasonographic or MRI depiction must demonstrate complete coaptation of the tendon ends with the ankle in 20 degrees of plantarflexion. This is an *obligatory* evaluation. The goal of surgery on the Achilles tendon is the complete coaptation of the tendon stumps; thus, the requirements for achieving a successful result must be the same for nonoperative management. If the diagnostic tools (ultrasound, MRI) reveal a persisting gapping of the tendon ends, nonsurgical treatment cannot be utilized, or the patient

has to be informed that this treatment may lead to a higher risk of rerupture or result in a weak gastroc-soleus muscle unit.

2. Because nonoperative treatment offers no method of mechanically stabilizing the tendon stumps, gapping is possible as the patient becomes increasingly mobile. Therefore, a sonographic verification is required after 4 weeks of treatment to verify normal tendon apposition and healing. Clinically, at that stage the restoration of the continuity of the tendon should be palpable. When performing minor ankle plantarflexion against resistance, the physician should feel a slight tensioning of the palpated gastrocnemius muscle. Ultrasonography will reveal the restored continuity of the tendon. Usually the tendon regeneration is sparse and appears as a nonhomogeneous structure with echogenic, hypogenic reflexes, and a width between 6 and 10 mm (normal width is 6 mm).

3. At 8 weeks, treatment with a protective orthotic device, therapy walker, or boots is stopped. Ultrasound imaging at this stage is obligatory to ensure that the tendon no longer needs protection. Just as every fracture's union is demonstrated by imaging studies before loading the bone, one should apply the same principle to the Achilles tendon.

4. Usually the regenerated tendon at this stage has become larger with a tendon width of 10 to 14 mm. On ultrasonography, a more structural alignment of the fibers will be apparent. Clinically, a broad, stable tendon is palpable, the Thompson test is negative, and in plantarflexion the patient can exert moderate power against resistance. If a sparse regenerate with an hourglass appearance at the former rupture site is palpable, an MRI or ultrasonography by an experienced radiologist is obligatory, as tendon healing probably is incomplete. Ultrasonographic examination will also show an hourglass narrowing of the tendon without hypogenic regenerate tissue.

5. Gapping of the tendon stumps, apparent by ultrasound images at 4 weeks, means that the tendon will heal with elongation. So, if there are no contraindications to surgical intervention, a percutaneous suture of the Achilles tendon should be performed at this point. The treatment in the orthosis/boot is then resumed for another 8 weeks with the standard sonographic controls. Gapping after 8 weeks has the same consequences as described above. A poor regenerate with restoration of the continuity means delayed healing and requires prolonged protection for 2 to 4 additional weeks. In our prospective sonographic study, we have found an increase of the regenerated tendon in the functional treatment from the 6th to the 12th week with a maximum occurring at the 10th week (Fig. 5.2). In medically compromised patients (e.g., with a spontaneous rupture after heart or kidney transplantation), we have seen a regeneration of the tendon at 6 months, where the patients have been protected by a therapy boot.

Treatment Plan

The Variostabil© (Orthotech GmbH, 82131 Gauting, Germany, http://www.orthotech-gmbh.de) boot plays a major role at our rehabilitation center for the regaining of functional performance of the Achilles unit. The concept of this boot is to prevent stress at the Achilles rupture site, while allowing axial loading, which promotes safe and powerful tendon healing (Fig. 5.3).

The boot has a plastic tongue to prevent ankle dorsiflexion; the lateral shaft-stabilization reduces torsion, and the reducible heel pad allows a gradual

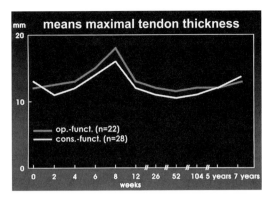

Fig. 5.2. Means of maximal tendon thickness in a prospective, randomized, 7-year follow-up study comparing monoperative with operative treatment

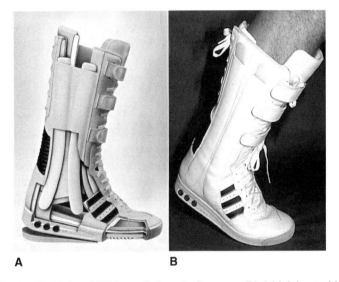

A   **B**

Fig. 5.3. (A) The Variostabil© boot; Orthotech, Germany. (B) A high boot with lateral stabilization, reducible heel (2 cm) and a stiff dorsal tongue to prevent dorsiflexion

adjustment from 20 degrees of plantarflexion to a neutral position. The functional concept of this boot, which was to allow protected gastrocnemius activities, was proven by electromyography, which demonstrated comparable amplitudes to the uninjured side after 3 months of treatment.[14] With a properly fitted boot, the patient is allowed to initiate walking with full weight bearing and to continue doing so as limited by pain and swelling. Thus, the patient may quickly return to performing normal daily activities.

Rehabilitation with the Therapy Boot (First 8 Weeks)

Initial treatment after tendon rupture is directed toward minimizing pain and swelling by use of analgesics and nonsteroidal antiinflammatory drugs (NSAIDs). The patient is protected in a plaster splint in the equinus position if the variostabie © boot is not immediately available. With the boot, the patient is allowed to walk with full weight bearing as quickly as the patient's pain will allow. For 6 weeks, the therapy boot is worn 24 hours a day (although the patient can wear a plaster splint overnight if desired). For an additional 2 weeks, the boot is worn only during the daytime.

At 2 to 3 weeks after injury, the patient may use a stationary bicycle, but only by exerting hind-foot pressure to move the pedals and only with a light application of power. Self-applied proprioceptive training with one-leg-stand stabilization exercises in the boot (the patient stands on the operative leg in the boot and tries to balance) should be performed daily.

In ambitious patients, after 4 weeks, physiotherapy is allowed with strengthening exercises (isometric exercises, isokinetic bicycle), proprioceptive neuromuscular facilitation (PNF), and coordination exercises in the boot. In addition, ultrasound application (1 MHz) and cryotherapy are performed to enhance tendon regeneration. From the sixth week on, leg-press training is begun in the boot.

After 8 weeks, an ultrasonographic examination evaluates the restoration of tendon continuity and confirms regeneration. If the patient has achieved an appropriate tendon regeneration (usually by 8 to 12 weeks, which should be confirmed by MRI or sonography), the treatment in the boot is discontinued. A small 1-cm heel lift placed in the normal shoe is recommended for a further 6 to 8 weeks. Jogging is allowed after 3 months if the patient's coordination and muscle power is appropriate.

Rehabilitation Following Boot Protection (9 to 12 Weeks)

The first treatment goal, after completion of protected treatment in the boot, is to have the patient regain coordination and proprioception. The limb is weakened at the gastroc-soleus muscle and the tendon regenerate's ultimate tensile strength cannot resist maximal uncontrolled dorsiflexion of the ankle, which could happen unintentionally, such as by slipping off a step or stepping in a hole. In the functional boot treatment, in contrast to cast immobilization treatment, these essential qualities can be trained in a therapy boot or appropriate orthosis from the very beginning. This is an advantage when we start the rehab without protective means.

Muscle strengthening is begun in a concentric (plantarflexion) mode because it minimizes the stress on the tendon regenerate, which is "moldable" and can lengthen at this early stage. That is why *passive* dorsiflexion by a physiotherapist is dangerous and not allowed. Shortening of the Achilles tendon is a minor problem only seen in operatively treated patients. A lengthened Achilles tendon with weak push-off is a tremendous problem (Fig. 5.4) and cannot be treated conservatively.

Strengthening is begun by having the patient perform double heel rises on a daily basis; this way, the uninjured leg helps the injured side recover. A step walker, cross trainer, and stationary bike provide additional exercise for the daily rehabilitation program. The patient must be aware that physiotherapy is only a "coaching" and "fine-tuning" activity toward regaining strength, coordination, and proprioception. The onus of exercises is accomplished through a daily workout by the patient himself. In untrained and obese patients, gymnastics in an indoor or outdoor pool using the buoyant force of water is extremely helpful to overcome the primary weakness of the calf muscles. After regaining

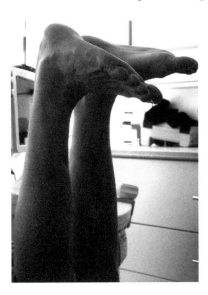

Fig. 5.4. A lengthened Achilles tendon with increased dorsiflexion

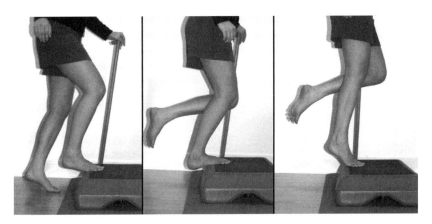

Fig. 5.5. After regaining calf muscle power, daily single leg heel rise (three sets of 15) and dorsiflexion on a stair can be performed for at least 8 to 12 months to improve calf muscle power

calf muscle power, such that the patient can perform 15 double heel rises three times a day, single-leg dorsiflexion and plantarflexion on a stair can be initiated and must continue for at least 8 to 12 months (Fig. 5.5).

From our experience and research, tensile resistance to maximum strain is achieved about 6 months after surgery. At that stage, tendon thickness, according to our sonographic studies, reaches about 2.5 to three times normal size (16 to 20 mm), which enables an appropriate stability to resist a force of three to five times body weight.

Jogging and low-impact activities are now allowed when the healed tendon regenerate is 12 to 14 mm after 4 to 5 months, implying stable coordinative and proprioceptive capacities. Regaining maximal performance requires at least 1 year of exercises.

In competitive athletes, a new-generation-type of kinesio taping (Leukotape © K, BSN medical, Hamburg, Germany) is helpful to support function and give the athlete more confidence in the stability of the Achilles tendon.

Complications

Poor Regenerate

Tendon healing usually follows a predictable pattern, but in our practice about 2% to 3% of the patients experience poor tendon regenerates, seen during sonographic follow-up examinations at between 4 and 8 weeks (Fig. 5.6). This is predictable in some cases where fibroblast-inhibiting agents such as cortisone are used or other general catabolic diseases exist that effect tendon healing. Usually, the regenerate has thickened significantly after 6 to 8 weeks, so that the real problem arises at the 8-week sonographic (but also clinical) control. Improving vascularity by ultrasound application (1 MHz) or via moist heat twice a day normally resolves this problem within 2 to 3 weeks. Protection with the therapy boot has to be prolonged over the 8-week period without reducing the mobility and activity that has already been obtained. In cases with an hourglass phenomenon (a palpable small dint in the tendon), the indication for a percutaneous suture should be indicated amply (Fig. 5.7). Surgical intervention means another 8 weeks in the orthosis or therapy boot.

Rerupture

As tendon healing is normally not demonstrated either by ultrasound or MRI, especially in the nonoperative treatment, the rerupture rate is certainly higher for nonoperative patients[15] (about 4% to 6%) compared with operative treatment (my personal rerupture rate, applying my follow-up protocol, is 2%). A biologic problem that underlies the reruptures is a different elasticity modulus between the normal tendon and the regenerate. To my personal experience, a rerupture nearly never occurs at the same area; in distal rupture sites it happens more proximally, and in proximal sites more distally. Tendon healing

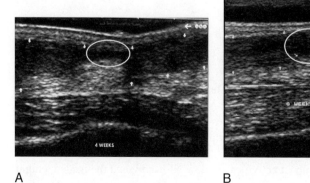

A   B

Fig. 5.6. (A) Sparse regenerate with hourglass phenomenon after 4 weeks. (B) Sparse regenerate with hourglass phenomenon after 8 weeks

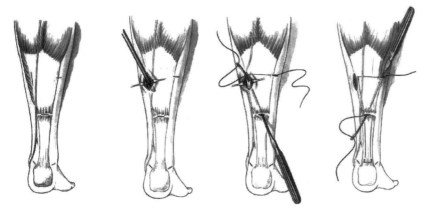

Fig. 5.7. Percutaneous suture according to Paessler. (From Thermann H. Neue Techniken. Fußchirurgie. Steinkopff Verlag Darmstadt, 2004:2–4, with permission of Springer Science and Business Media Heidelberg, Germany)

is comparable to connecting two tubes with a bushing. At the proximal and distal sides, we have rather normal tendons as the regenerate site is bigger and adherent to the surrounding tissue. In other words, the regenerated tendon is stiffer than the normal tendon,

If a major force is activated (recruitment of all muscle fibers, unintended maximal dorsiflexion), the junction between the stiff regenerate and the normal tendon is the weakest link and has a limited expansion before rupturing.

Reruptures can occur in the plaster or in the boot at any time, but mostly between the eighth and 14th week after the initial rupture.

Rupture morphology is crucial for planning further treatment. If during sonography, a gap is visible between the tendon stumps in plantarflexion, a percutaneous suture should be performed.

A sparse regenerate at the reruptured site also requires surgical adaptation of the stumps by percutaneous suture, as this technique does not deleteriously effect the newly rebuilt vascularity that enables healing of the renewed tendon.

Utilizing the biology of tendon healing, combined with minimally invasive surgery to provide stabilization of the tendon stumps during the initial treatment and healing, would seem to give a distinct advantage to the percutaneous surgical technique described by Buchgraber and Paessler.[16] Using only five small incisions, a 1.3-mm PDS cord is guided percutaneously by means of an awl. It connects the proximal tendon with the calcaneal insertion and crosses the rupture site, thereby acting as an internal fixator. To tighten the cord into the tendon, multiple dorsiflexions of the foot are performed. Another advantage of this technique is that it retains the remaining integrity of the paratendon, which is essentially important for the healing process. To prevent the potential risk of injuring the sural nerve, an endoscopically assisted percutaneous technique with a 2.8-mm arthroscope can be used.[9]

Hypertrophic tendon regeneration at the rupture site is comparable to the way in which a bone fracture mends itself and has a tremendous potential for healing, if stability is guaranteed. It is up to the experience and the preferences of the surgeon whether to proceed with nonoperative treatment or to shift (especially if the patient requests this) to a percutaneous suture. A rerupture requires the patient to undergo the entire treatment all over again.

The validity of this method, compared with operative treatment, could be proven in a series of more than 550 patients using a high shaft shoe, comparable to a modified boxer boot (Variostabil; Fig. 5.3).[17]

The indication for primary functional treatment, independent of the ultrasonographic or MRI findings, is not the elderly non-active patient or in patients with altered operation risk or reduced capacity for tissue regeneration (e.g., after organ transplantation surgery, systemic corticosteroid treatment, diabetes, etc.).[14] There is a clear preference for treatment in cases in which the tendon ends are virtually together. But in cases with considerable gapping, minimally invasive techniques (i.e., percutaneous sutures) should be applied for tendon reconstruction, followed by a functional treatment in an appropriate orthosis. Even in generally compromised patients, a percutaneous suture is possible using local anesthesia and in a lateral position.

Evidence-Based Medicine

There are many meta-analyses of Achilles tendon rupture,[7,15,18–20] but most never consider coaptation of the tendon stumps as a fundamental criteria for comparison of surgical and nonsurgical treatments. Of course, we can compare everything, but then it is not unexpected when nonoperative treatment results in more reruptures (about 6%) and reduced tendon power in the functional test.

We have performed a prospective randomized study with 7 years of follow-up comparing nonoperative with operative treatment. Both groups have had identical after-treatments (therapy boot) and sonographic and MRI assessments (adaptation of the tendon stumps, at 4 weeks, 8 weeks, 6 months, 12 months, 2 years, and 7 years of follow-up). Utilizing a 100-point scoring system[17,21] and power measurement, we could not find significant differences, which underscores that applying these criteria, one can achieve identical results (Fig. 5.8).

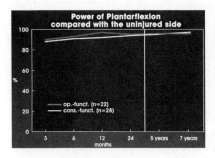

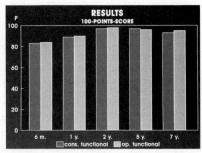

A   B

Fig. 5.8. (A) Results of calf muscle strength measurement in a prospective, randomized, 7-year follow-up study. (B) Results of 100–point scoring system in a prospective, randomized, 7-year follow-up study

Operative Treatment

Issues that might force the decision for operative treatment include the following:

- Patients with poor compliance for primary functional treatment, such as alcoholics or drug addicts
- Patients who insist on, or feel safer with, a surgical procedure
- Patients in whom no coaptation of the tendon stumps was found sonographically or on MRI
- Patients with a demonstrable disruption of the soleus muscle
- Patients, such as top athletes, for whom surgery is intended for retention of the gastroc-soleus-Achilles complex to achieve an optimal lever arm for push off. (The Lace technique by Segesser pays special attention to the rotation of radiating tendon bundles, as described by Cummins. With his technique, Segesser provides an adequate reinsertion of the medial gastrocnemius and soleus fibers, which are often disrupted or retracted in Achilles tendon ruptures in top-level athletes [Fig. 5.9].)
- Patients with distal ruptures (≤2 cm) near the calcaneal insertion, since plantarflexion usually does not allow approximation of the stumps
- Patients with avulsion or tendon laceration at the calcaneal insertion

Timing

It is generally possible to appose the tendon stumps within 3 to 5 weeks after rupture. In older ruptures, the tendon ends are usually retracted and need reconstructive modalities with gastroc-soleus mobilization to reduce the gap.

Conclusion

Nonoperative treatment of acute Achilles tendon rupture is a sophisticated specific therapy that requires strict indications to achieve a successful result. Most of the published studies do not fulfill these criteria, so an objective

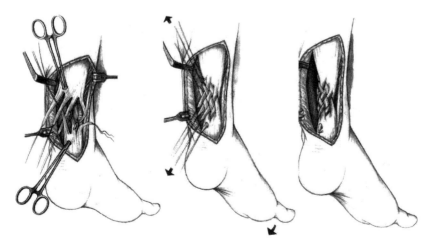

Fig. 5.9. The lace technique by Segesser. (From Thermann H. Neue Techniken. Fußchirurgie. Steinkopff Verlag Darmstadt, 2004:8–9, with permission of Springer Science and Business Media Heidelberg, Germany)

comparison with results of surgical treatment (where the tendon stumps always have a complete coaptation) is, from an absolute scientific point of view, not possible.

The goal of treatment today is not only the restoration of the tendon continuity, but also the regaining of the patient's former activity level at the earliest possible time. This not only is achievable by both appropriate operative and nonoperative techniques, but also depends on an adequate after-treatment and rehabilitation protocol with tendon healing controls.

References

1. Christensen J. Rupture Achilles tendon. Acta Chir Scand 1953;106(50).
2. Schonbauer HR. [Diseases of the Achilles tendon]. Wien Klin Wochenschr Suppl 1986;168:1–47.
3. Thermann H. Treatment of Achilles tendon ruptures. Foot Ankle Clin 1999;4(4):773–87.
4. Cetti R, Christensen SE, Ejsted R, et al. Operative versus nonoperative treatment of Achilles tendon rupture. A prospective randomized study and review of the literature. Am J Sports Med 1993;21(6):791–9.
5. Inglis AE, Scuco TP. Surgical repair of ruptures of the tendo Achillis. Clin Orthop 1981;156:160–9.
6. Jacobs D, Martens M, Van Audekercke R, et al. Comparison of conservative and operative treatment of Achilles tendon rupture. Am J Sports Med 1978;6(3):107–11.
7. Lo IK, Kirkley A, Nonweiler B, et al. Operative versus nonoperative treatment of acute Achilles tendon ruptures: a quantitative review. Clin J Sport Med 1997;7(3):207–11.
8. Nistor L. Surgical and non-surgical treatment of Achilles Tendon rupture. A prospective randomized study. J Bone Joint Surg [Am] 1981;63(3):394–9.
9. Thermann H. [Treatment of Achilles tendon rupture]. Unfallchirurg 1998;101(4): 299–314.
10. Jozsa L, Kvist M, Balint BJ, et al. The role of recreational sport activity in Achilles tendon rupture. A clinical, pathoanatomical, and sociological study of 292 cases. Am J Sports Med 1989;17(3):338–43.
11. Riede D. [Comments on "Therapy and late results of subcutaneous Achilles tendon rupture"]. Beitr Orthop Traumatol 1972;19(6):328–31.
12. Arner O, Lindholm A. Subcutaneous rupture of the Achilles tendon; a study of 92 cases. Acta Chir Scand Suppl 1959;116(suppl 239):1–51.
13. Kannus P, Jozsa L. Histopathological changes preceding spontaneous rupture of a tendon. A controlled study of 891 patients. J Bone Joint Surg [Am] 1991;73(10):1507–1525.
14. Thermann H. [Rupture of the Achilles tendon—conservative functional treatment]. Z Orthop Ihre Grenzgeb 1998;136(5):Oa20–2.
15. Khan RJ, Fick D, Keogh A, et al. Treatment of acute Achilles tendon ruptures. A meta-analysis of randomized, controlled trials. J Bone Joint Surg [Am] 2005;87(10):2202–10.
16. Buchgraber A, Paessler HH. Percutaneous repair of Achilles tendon rupture. Immobilization versus functional postoperative treatment. Clin Orthop 1997;341:113–22.
17. Thermann H, Zwipp H, Tscherne H. [Functional treatment concept of acute rupture of the Achilles tendon. 2 years results of a prospective randomized study]. Unfallchirurg 1995;98(1):21–32.
18. Bhandari M, Guyatt GH, Siddiqui F, et al. Treatment of acute Achilles tendon ruptures: a systematic overview and metaanalysis. Clin Orthop Rel Res 2002;(400):190–200.

19. Dobson MH, Nguyen C. Treatment of acute Achilles tendon ruptures. A meta-analysis of randomized, controlled trials. J Bone Joint Surg [Am] 2005;87(10):1160.
20. McCormack RG. Treatment of acute Achilles tendon ruptures: a systematic overview and metaanalysis. Clin J Sport Med 2003;13(3):194.
21. McComis GP, Nawoczenski DA, DeHaven KE. Functional bracing for rupture of the Achilles tendon. Clinical results and analysis of ground-reaction forces and temporal data. J Bone Joint Surg [Am] 1997;79(12):1799–808.

6

Acute Repairs of the Achilles Tendon by the Percutaneous Technique

Ansar Mahmood and Nicola Maffulli

Despite being the strongest tendon in the human body, the Achilles tendon is the most commonly ruptured.[1,2] Among physicians, there is considerable debate surrounding the etiopathogenesis and the management of acute ruptures. Such injuries commonly occur in the occasional athlete and middle-aged men. The following case study is an example of a typical patient who presented to our outpatient clinic.

Case Study

A 38-year-old, self-employed computer software engineer, who played soccer once a week, attended the Fracture Clinic 2 days following an injury to his right Achilles tendon (AT). While participating in a soccer match, he pushed off on his left foot and felt something give at the back of his ankle. This resulted in acute severe pain, and he was unable to bear weight or drive home following the injury. At the Accident Unit, he was radiographed, and a clinical suspicion of Achilles tendon rupture was formulated.

The patient was otherwise fit and well, took no regular medication, and was a nonsmoker. There was no family medical history of note, and he had no previous similar injuries.

On examination, he was unable to stand unassisted, and could not stand on his toes. There was swelling and bruising around the posterior ankle, and dependent swelling in the foot. The foot was held in about the mid-equinus position.

The patient was asked to lie prone on the examination couch, where gentle palpation revealed a palpable gap, consistent with a tear in the AT (Fig. 6.1) . The Simmonds and Thompson calf squeeze test[3] was performed on both legs for comparison, and a readily appreciable difference in the degree of plantarflexion was noted. The injured foot did not move on a gentle squeeze of the calf, whereas the normal side showed ankle plantarflexion (Figs. 6.2 and 6.3) .

The patient was then asked to actively flex his knees to 90 degrees. The left foot fell into neutral in comparison to the unaffected side. This is the Matles test,[4] where a degree of plantarflexion is maintained on the normal side by the intact AT (Fig.6.4) .

J.A. Nunley (ed.), *The Achilles Tendon: Treatment and Rehabilitation*, DOI: 10.1007/978-1-387-79206-4_6, © Springer Science+Business Media, LLC 2009

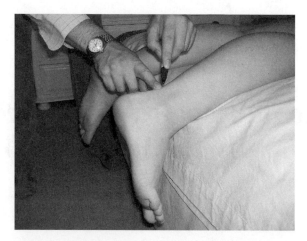

Fig. 6.1. Finger indicating palpable gap

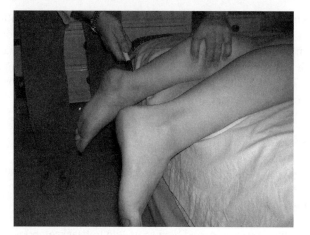

Fig. 6.2. Thompson test: intact Achilles tendon, etc. leads to plantarflexion of the left foot on calf squeeze

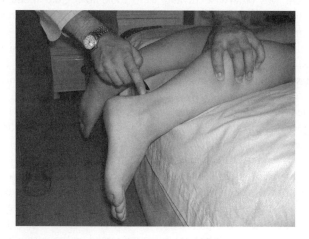

Fig. 6.3. Thompson test: no plantar flexion on calf squeeze of the right foot due to a ruptured Achilles tendon

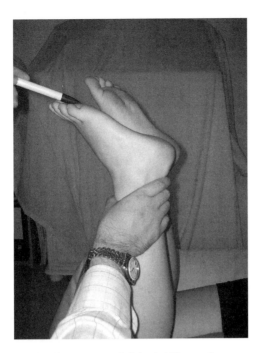

Fig. 6.4. Matles test, showing a ruptured right Achilles tendon

Once clinical confirmation was made of an acute rupture of the AT, the patient was counseled regarding the different modes of treatment, namely conservative (nonoperative) and open versus percutaneous repair. The patient opted for percutaneous repair of his Achilles tendon under local anesthesia. Our technique is described in detail below.

Imaging

If the diagnosis is in doubt, then imaging can assist in establishing the existence of a rupture. However, this is not our routine practice, as it adds little to the management of the patient.

Ultrasound scans[5] or magnetic resonance imaging[6] helps to confirm the diagnosis in specific cases (usually chronic ruptures). Ultrasonography reveals an acoustic vacuum between the tendon edges. Magnetic resonance imaging reveals generalized high signal intensity on T2-weighted images. On T1-weighted images, the rupture appears as a disruption of the signal within the tendon substance.

Conservative Management

Excellent results have been reported with conservative management using a hard cast for 1 month before switching to a functional brace for an additional 1 month.[7]

However, it has also been shown that rerupture rates can be unacceptably high in some patients—from about 10% to 20%.[8-10] In contrast, following surgical management rerupture is usually reported at around 2% to 3%.[9,11]

Nonoperative management may also lengthen the tendon, altering its function.[12] Secondary surgical correction may then be required,[13] and can be avoided with primary surgery.

Open Repair

Surgical management significantly reduces the risk of Achilles tendon rerupture, but increases the risk of infection when compared with conservative management.[14]

Arner and Lindholm,[15] in their series of 86 operative repairs, reported a 24% complication rate, including one death from pulmonary embolism. Lo et al[10] reported that open repair induces 20 times more minor to moderate complications than conservative management, with no significant difference for major complications.

Numerous methods have been described for open repair, from simple end-to-end repair (Bunnell/Kessler) to complex techniques involving tendon grafting and fascial reinforcement. Thus far, one suture method has not shown itself to be superior to another for fresh ruptures.

The outcome of open repair has demonstrated a significant disparity from unit to unit.[15,16] These differences are likely to be multifactorial, and may well result from patient selection and compliance, as well as subtle variations in surgical technique from surgeon to surgeon, the type of suture material used, and the location of the incision.

Percutaneous Repair

Percutaneous repair is a compromise between open surgery and conservative management. The aim of percutaneous repair is to provide a better functional outcome than conservative management, with a similar functional outcome and rerupture rate to that of open repair, while minimizing patient dissatisfaction with some aspects of the open repair. Some techniques have been in use for 30 years.

Ma and Griffith[17] pioneered the technique with a reported excellent success rate with no reruptures and two minor complications.

The early reports outlined a possible increased risk of rerupture and of damage to the sural nerve. However, these studies were very heterogeneous with regard to selection, operative techniques and outcome measures. Some studies have demonstrated that the rate of rerupture is higher in percutaneous repair than after open procedures,[18,19] although these studies are now dated, and also do not compare like with like.

More recent studies comparing open and percutaneous repair show that the two repair techniques produce similar outcomes,[20] and advocate percutaneous repair over open techniques after concluding that percutaneous repair had a lower infection rate, was more cosmetically acceptable, and the functional results showed no significant difference.

Cretnik et al.[21] further expanded on the benefits of percutaneous repair and the controversy regarding the optimal management of the fresh total Achilles tendon ruptures. They concluded after at least a 2-year follow-up that there were significantly fewer major complications in the group of percutaneous repairs in comparison with the group of open repairs (p = .03), and a lower total number of complications (p = .013). There was no statistically significant difference in rates of rerupture and sural nerve entrapment. Functional assessment between the two groups was similar using the American Orthopaedic Foot and Ankle Society scale and the Holz score.

Techniques

Ma and Griffith[17] described a technique of percutaneous repair of the Achilles tendon using six stab incisions over the tendon in 18 patients. The suture was passed through the stab incisions, and crisscrossed through the tendon. They reported one incidence of sensory disturbance and one patient with sural nerve entrapment.

Webb and Bannister[22] described a percutaneous technique that medializes the proximal incision to keep away from the sural nerve.

McClelland and Maffulli[23] described a percutaneous technique of repair of ruptured Achilles tendons similar to that described by Webb and Bannister, but using a Kessler-type suture.

We now perform percutaneous repair of Achilles tendon rupture using a minimally invasive procedure with five small incisions, four of which are 1 cm long, and the fifth being 2 cm.

Preoperative Planning

Once the diagnosis is made, the patient needs a full preoperative assessment to investigate, manage and control any comorbidities.

The preoperative functional status should be recorded and the neurovascular status of the affected limb should be documented. Particular attention should be paid to the status of the sural nerve.

We recommend deep vein thrombosis (DVT) prophylaxis as per local protocol. However, we do not routinely use DVT prophylaxis in athletes.

An equinus back slab is sometimes used for preoperative comfort.

Valid written consent is obtained by the operating surgeon. Sural nerve damage, rerupture, infection, and impaired function should be discussed with the patient, including alternative management strategies and their outcomes.

Operation: Technique

Local anesthesia infiltration is used. A 50:50 mixture of 10 mL of 2% lignocaine hydrochloride (Antigen Pharmaceuticals Ltd., Roscrea, Ireland) and 10 mL of 0.25% bupivacaine hydrochloride (Astra Pharmaceuticals Ltd., Kings Langley, England) is instilled into an area of between 8 and 10 cm around the ruptured Achilles tendon.

The patient is placed in the prone position, and a pillow is placed beneath the anterior aspect of the ankles to allow the feet to hang free. The operating table is angled down approximately 20 degrees cranially to reduce venous pooling in the feet and ankles.

The affected leg is prepared with antiseptic. We do not use a tourniquet.

Five stab incisions are made over the Achilles tendon (Fig. 6.5) . The first is directly over the palpable defect, and is approximately 2 cm in a transverse

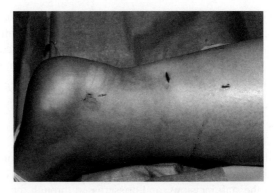

Fig. 6.5. The five stab incisions around the Achilles tendon rupture

direction. The other incisions are about 4 cm proximal and 4 cm distal to the first incision, and are vertical 1-cm stab incisions on the medial and lateral aspect of the Achilles tendon.

We advocate blunt dissection with a small hemostat directly onto the Achilles tendon, and therefore avoid damaging the sural nerve, which crosses the lateral border of the Achilles tendon about 10 cm proximal to its insertion into the calcaneus.[24] A small hemostat is used to free the tendon sheath from the overlying subcutaneous tissue (Fig. 6.6) .

A 1 PDS II (Ethicon, Johnson and Johnson Intl., Brussels, Belgium) double-stranded suture on a long curved needle is passed transversely through the lateral proximal stab incision, passing through the substance of the tendon and out through the medial proximal stab incision (Fig. 6.7) .

The needle is then reintroduced into the medial proximal stab incision through a different more proximal entry point in the tendon and passed longitudinally and distally through the tendon, to lock into the tendon. Finally, it is directed toward the middle incision and out through the ruptured tendon end.

The suture end still protruding from the lateral proximal stab incision is re-threaded onto the needle and reintroduced via the lateral proximal stab incision into the tendon substance through a more proximal entry point. It is also passed longitudinally and distally through the tendon to exit from the middle incision. Traction is applied to the suture to ensure a satisfactory grip within the tendon (Fig. 6.8) . If the suture pulls through, the procedure is repeated. We use an eight-stranded method by doubling the sutures used for the modified Kessler suturing technique we are describing.

The same procedure is carried out for the distal half of the ruptured tendon (Fig. 6.9) .

The sutures are then tied (Fig. 6.10) with the ankle in maximal plantar-flexion, and buried deep in the tendon using a hemostat (Fig. 6.11) . The skin wounds are closed with undyed subcuticular 3-0 Vicryl (Ethicon, Edinburgh, UK) suture, and nonadherent dressings are applied.

A full plaster of Paris cast is applied in the operating room with the ankle in maximal equinus. The cast is split on both medial and lateral sides to allow for swelling (Fig. 6.12) .

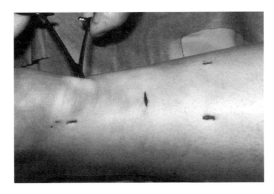

Fig. 6.6. Hemostat being used to free the Achilles from any subcutaneous and peritendinous adhesions

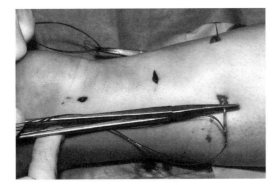

Fig. 6.7. Needle introduced into the lateral proximal stab incision through the substance of the tendon

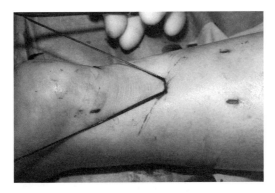

Fig. 6.8. Needle reintroduced into the medial proximal stab incision through a different entry point in the tendon and passed longitudinally and proximally through the tendon, directed toward the middle incision and out through the ruptured tendon end. The same is done with the suture protruding from the lateral proximal stab incision once it is re-threaded onto a needle. Traction is applied to the suture to ensure a satisfactory grip within the tendon

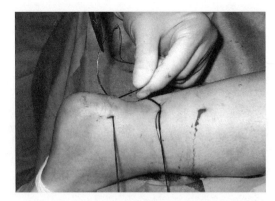

Fig. 6.9. The same procedure as in Figure 6.8 is repeated for the distal portion of the rupture

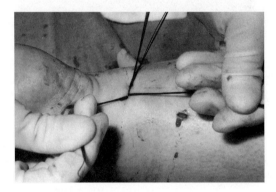

Fig. 6.10. The sutures are then tied with the ankle in physiologic plantarflexion

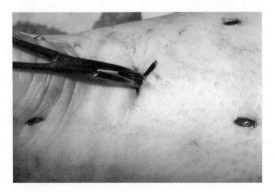

Fig. 6.11. A hemostat is used to bury the suture into the tissues

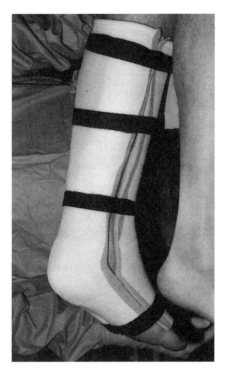

Fig. 6.12. A full plaster of Paris cast is applied in the operating room with the ankle in physiologic equinus. The cast is split on both medial and lateral sides to accommodate swelling

Complications

Hematomas can lead to infection and wound breakdown, especially in light of the tenuous blood supply to the Achilles tendon. In our practice, we have found this very infrequent, given the small incisions used. Infection is a recognized complication of the open approach, and is reduced with percutaneous techniques.[22,23]

Sural nerve damage can cause altered dermatomal sensation or a painful neuroma. Patients can experience anesthesia of the lateral aspect of the foot, and some report difficulty with shoes as a result of this. This can be avoided with blunt dissection directly onto the Achilles tendon and placement of the skin incision such that the sutures are distant from the sural nerve.

Rerupture is a documented complication. The use of modern suture materials with the number of intratendinous threads comparable to what is used in open repairs minimizes this complication.

More recent studies comparing percutaneous and open repair show similar results, with no difference in rerupture rate between the two repair techniques.[5] However, a significantly higher rate of infective wound complications result from using open repair.[20]

The clinician should be vigilant for DVT due to the patient being treated in a plaster cast and having an injury that prevents normal ambulation. It is appropriate to look for this problem whenever patients are examined out of cast, and managed appropriately if suspected. Early postoperative rehabilitation aims to reduce this risk.

Postoperative Management

The operated leg is elevated immediately postoperatively, and the patient's neurovascular status is documented. A physiotherapist should perform a review to ensure the patient is safe for discharge from the ambulation point of view.

A full cast is retained for 2 weeks, and the patient is able to bear weight as comfort allows. During the period in the cast, patients are advised to perform gentle isometric contractions of the gastroc-soleus complex, and elevate the limb when at rest.

At the 2-week review, the patient's wounds are inspected.

An anterior splint is worn with the foot plantarflexed for a further 4 weeks. While this is in situ, patients are advised to mobilize partial weight bearing, increasing to weight bearing as able by 4 weeks. In addition, patients are encouraged to invert and evert the foot and to plantar flex it against resistance on a regular basis.

Once the splint is removed, physiotherapy follow-up is arranged, initially for gentle mobilization. Light exercise can be started 2 weeks after cast removal. Patients should be fully weight bearing by that time.

References

1. Maffulli N. Rupture of the Achilles tendon. J Bone Joint Surg [Am] 1999;81A: 1019–36.
2. Jozsa L, Kvist M, Balint BJ, . The role of recreational sport activity in Achilles tendon rupture. A clinical, pathoanatomical, and sociological study of 292 cases. Am J Sports Med 1989;17(3):338–43.
3. Simmonds FA. The diagnosis of the ruptured Achilles tendon. Practitioner 1957;179:56–8.
4. Matles AL. Rupture of the tendo Achilles. Another diagnostic test. Bull Hosp Joint Dis 1975;36:48–51.
5. Maffulli N, Dymond NP, Capasso G. Ultrasonographic findings in subcutaneous rupture of Achilles tendon. J Sports Med Phys Fitness 1989;29(4):365–8.
6. Kabbani YM, Mayer DP. Magnetic resonance imaging of tendon pathology about the foot and ankle. Part I. Achilles tendon. J Am Podiatr Med Ass 1993;83:418–20.
7. Wallace RG, Traynor IE, Kernohan WG, et al. Combined conservative and orthotic management of acute ruptures of the Achilles tendon. J Bone Joint Surg [Am] 2004;86:1198–202.
8. Persson A, Wredmark T. The treatment of total ruptures of the Achilles tendon by plaster immobilisation. Int Orthop 1979;3:149–52.
9. Moller M, Movin T, Granhed H, et al. Acute rupture of tendon Achilles. A prospective randomised study of comparison between surgical and non-surgical treatment. J Bone Joint Surg [Br] 2001;83(6):843–8.
10. Lo IK, Kirkley A, Nonweiler B, et al. Operative versus nonoperative treatment of acute Achilles tendon ruptures: a quantitative review. Clin J Sports Med 1997;7: 207–11.
11. Wong J, Barrass V, Maffulli N. Quantitative review of operative and non-operative management of Achilles tendon ruptures. Am J Sports Med 2002;30:565–75.

12. Bohnsack M, Ruhmann O, Kirsch L, et al. Surgical shortening of the Achilles tendon for correction of elongation following healed conservatively treated Achilles tendon rupture. Z Orthop Ihre Grenzgeb 2000;138:501–5.
13. Soma C, Mandelbaum B. Repair of acute Achilles tendon ruptures. Orthop Clin North Am 1976;7:241–6.
14. Bhandari M, Guyatt GH, Siddiqui F, et al. Treatment of acute Achilles tendon ruptures: a systematic overview and meta-analysis. Clin Orthop 2002;400:190–200.
15. Arner O, Lindholm A. Subcutaneous rupture of the Achilles tendon. A study of 92 cases. Acta Chir Scand 1959;116(239):1–5.
16. Soldatis J, Goodfellow D, Wilber J. End to end operative repair of Achilles tendon rupture. Am J Sports Med 1997;25:90–5.
17. Ma GWC, Griffith TG. Percutaneous repair of acute closed ruptures Achilles tendon. A new technique. Clin Orthop 1977;128:247–55.
18. Aracil J, Lozano J, Torro V, et al. Percutaneous suture of Achilles tendon ruptures. Foot Ankle 1992;13:350–1.
19. Bradley J, Tibone J. Percutaneous and open surgical repairs of Achilles tendon ruptures. A comparative study. Am J Sports Med 1990;18:188–95.
20. Lim J, Dalal R, Waseem M. Percutaneous vs. open repair of the ruptured Achilles tendon—a prospective randomized controlled study. Foot Ankle Int 2001;22(7):559–68.
21. Cretnik A, Kosanovic M, Smrkolj V. Percutaneous versus open repair of the ruptured Achilles tendon: a comparative study. Am J Sports Med 2005;33(9):1369–79.
22. Webb JM, Bannister GC. Percutaneous repair of the ruptured tendo Achilles. J Bone Joint Surg [Br] 1999;81(5):877–80.
23. McClelland D, Maffulli N. Percutaneous repair of ruptured Achilles tendon. J R Coll Surg Edinb 2002;41:613–8.
24. Webb J, Moorjani N, Radford M. Anatomy of the sural nerve and its relation to the Achilles tendon. Foot Ankle Int 2000;21(6):475–7.

7

Mini-Open Repair of Acute Ruptures

Mathieu Assal

Though an increasing number of reports in the recent literature tend to favor operative treatment of a fresh rupture of the Achilles tendon,[1–12] the exact type of operative procedure and the postoperative regimen remain controversial. Many investigators favor a formal operative approach to secure the best possible repair with the least chance of rerupture. Soft tissue concerns have led others to plan such a procedure only for the professional or high-level athlete, while planning a percutaneous procedure for others.[3,6] Ma and Griffith[13] developed such a technique and reported good results in 18 patients. However, there appear to be two problems with their approach. One is its potential for sural nerve injury. And two, since there is no open incision as the tendon ends are brought into apposition, the quality of the repair cannot be confirmed visually.

It is our belief that the best treatment is an operative one, and we were initially attracted to the method described by Kakiuchi[14] combining the advantages of the open and percutaneous techniques. To improve this technique, I developed a new instrument and surgical technique based on a cadaver study and led a prospective multicenter study[15] of the first 87 patients consecutively treated in this fashion, which included an early functional rehabilitation program. Following the very good results, we made this procedure our operation of choice for acute Achilles tendon ruptures.

Materials

Cadaver Study

A new instrument was designed based on the morphology of the distal triceps muscle and Achilles tendon. In 16 fresh cadaver legs, we specifically looked at the mean V-shaped angle and the mean surface of the tendon, that is, the transverse surface at the thinnest part of the tendon. We found that the mean V-shaped angle was 8 degrees and the mean transverse surface was 81 mm^2. With this information, we developed an instrument (Achillon®, Newdeal SA, Lyon, France) that conformed to the local anatomy. In these same cadaveric specimens, we created a transverse laceration of the Achilles tendon 4 cm above the calcaneal tuberosity and passed the new instrument according to

J.A. Nunley (ed.), *The Achilles Tendon: Treatment and Rehabilitation*,
DOI: 10.1007/978-1-387-79206-4_7, © Springer Science+Business Media, LLC 2009

the surgical procedure described below. Then we dissected each limb and modified our instrument based on the local anatomy of the muscle and tendon. Sutures were introduced by blunt needle, three proximal and three distal to the laceration site. There was no conflict between the instrument branches, and the needles and the sutures were not macroscopically damaged by the instrument. In all cases the sutures were found beneath the paratenon without strangulation of the tendon. We did not notice any entrapment of the sural nerve in the sutures, no macroscopic injury to the sural nerve, and no evidence of disruption of the nerve sheath.

Instrument

The Achillon is made of a rigid polymer and designed to guide the passage of the sutures. It is composed of a pair of internal branches connected to a pair of external branches, with each branch having a line of apertures at the same level to allow easy and accurate passage of the sutures through all four branches (Fig. 7.1). The two internal branches are at an 8-degree angle to each other, following the V-shaped anatomic form of the tendon. A micrometric screw allows for varying the opening of the branches according to tendon morphology. A straight needle with its attached suture is used with a needle driver, designed to provide a larger support surface to push the needle through the soft tissues and at the same time protect the surgeon by preventing possible perforation of the glove from the end of the needle.

Operative Technique

The patient is placed in the prone position on the operating table with a tourniquet around the upper thigh. Both legs are included in the prep and drape

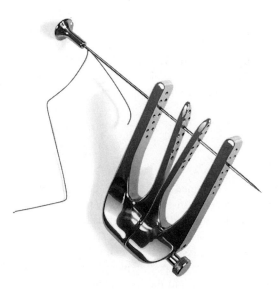

Fig. 7.1. The Achillon® instrument, with a straight needle and suture passed through one level of holes. (From Assal et al.,[15] with permission from the *Journal of Bone and Joint Surgery,* Inc.)

in order to compare Achilles tendon tension and spontaneous plantarflexion intraoperatively. Plastic drape is not used, and all patients receive antibiotic prophylaxis. The site of injury, represented by the gap or soft spot, is palpated. The incision is paratendinous and medial (Fig. 7.2) , beginning at the soft spot and extending approximately 2.0 cm proximally. The skin and subcutaneous tissue is gently retracted with hooks, and the paratenon is identified. The sheath is carefully opened, and each edge is tagged with a stay suture (Fig. 7.3) . Both stumps of the ruptured tendon are identified (Fig. 7.4) , and the exact site of rupture is carefully noted. The Achillon is introduced in the closed position under the paratenon in a proximal direction, with the tendon stump held with a small clamp under the instrument (Fig. 7.5) . The tendon stump is located between the two internal branches. As the instrument is introduced, it is progressively widened, holding the tendon stump firmly with the clamp. The position

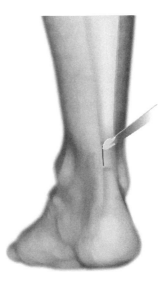

Fig. 7.2. Illustration of the skin incision, begun at the gap or soft spot, paratendinous and medial, and extended 1.5 to 2 cm proximally. (From Assal et al.,[15] with permission from the *Journal of Bone and Joint Surgery,* Inc.)

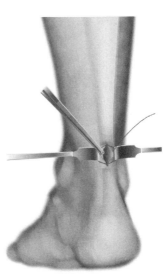

Fig. 7.3. The sheath opened longitudinally in the midline and a stay suture in place. (From Assal et al.,[15] with permission from the *Journal of Bone and Joint Surgery,* Inc.)

Fig. 7.4. The forceps grasping the proximal tendon stump. (From Assal et al.,[15] with permission from the *Journal of Bone and Joint Surgery,* Inc.)

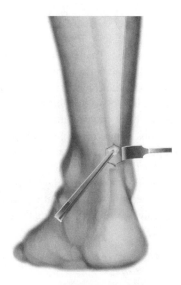

Fig. 7.5. Illustration showing the introduction of the instrument proximally under the paratenon. (From Assal et al.,[15] with permission from the *Journal of Bone and Joint Surgery,* Inc.)

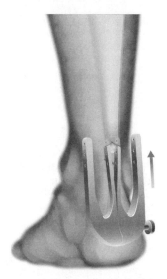

of the guide is confirmed by external palpation, and the surgeon should feel the tendon between the central (internal) branches of the instrument.

Three sutures are now passed from lateral to medial, usually beginning with the most proximal hole of the instrument (Fig. 7.6) . The end of each suture is held with a small clamp to keep them separate from each other. The instrument is then slowly withdrawn while progressively closing the branches. This maneuver results in the sutures sliding from an extracutaneous position to a peritendinous position; thus the tendon itself is the only tissue held by the sutures (Fig. 7.7) . Traction is applied to the three suture pairs to ensure their firm anchoring in the tendon, and they are individually clamped to prevent any confusion. The same sequence is performed on the distal stump with the instrument being introduced under the tendon sheath and pushed until it touches the calcaneum. All the sutures are now organized for tightening (Fig. 7.8) , which is

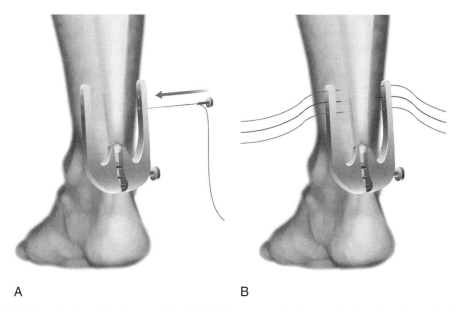

A   B

Fig. 7.6. (A) Introduction of the first needle. (B) All three sutures in the proximal tendon. (From Assal et al.,[15] with permission from the *Journal of Bone and Joint Surgery,* Inc.)

Fig. 7.7. The instrument being withdrawn, bringing the sutures from an extracutaneous to a peritendinous position. (From Assal et al.,[15] with permission from the *Journal of Bone and Joint Surgery,* Inc.)

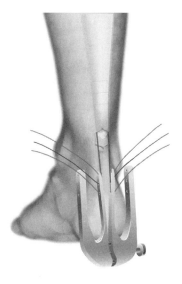

carried out with corresponding pairs, and the tendon reduction is under direct visual control (Fig. 7.9). If it is difficult to ascertain tendon length and reduction because the ends are too frayed, the tendon tension should be compared to that in the opposite leg. The tendon sheath is closed, and then the skin is closed with intradermal sutures. No drain is used, and a splint is applied holding the ankle in 30 degrees of flexion prior to moving or waking the patient. Low-molecular-weight heparin (subcutaneous administration) is used for prophylactic anticoagulation in all patients for 3 weeks postoperatively.

Fig. 7.8. The sutures organized for tightening. (From Assal et al.,[15] with permission from the *Journal of Bone and Joint Surgery,* Inc.)

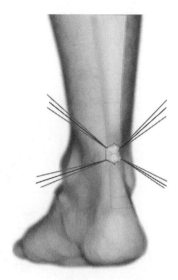

Fig. 7.9. The tendon reduction performed under direct vision, confirming apposition of the tendon ends. (From Assal et al.,[15] with permission from the *Journal of Bone and Joint Surgery,* Inc.)

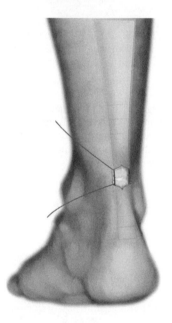

Rehabilitation Protocol

We instituted an early functional rehabilitation program, carefully supervised by a physical therapist, which is divided into four distinct stages. For the first 2 weeks, patients are allowed partial weight bearing (30 to 45 pounds) and maintained in the splint, full-time. Then gentle ankle range of motion (flexion and extension) is begun, as well as thigh muscle exercises and the use of a stationary bicycle. The goal is to reach a neutral ankle position by the end of the third week. After 3 weeks, full weight bearing is allowed with continuous use of the protective splint. At the end of 8 weeks, the splint is discontinued and weight bearing is allowed without any external support. A more intensive program of ankle range of motion, stretching, isometric, and proprioceptive exercises is instituted. Jogging is allowed at 3 months and more demanding sports at 6 months.

Case Study

A 35-year-old man presented to the emergency room 24 hours after sustaining an injury to his right ankle. While reaching for a difficult shot at tennis he felt a "pop" in the back of the ankle. He was able to walk, albeit with moderate pain. Physical examination revealed moderate swelling about the posterior aspect of the right ankle and foot. With the patient prone, spontaneous excess dorsiflexion of the right ankle was noted (Fig. 7.10) . A tender palpable defect was present in the Achilles tendon 4 cm proximal to its insertion (Fig. 7.11) . The Thompson test was positive (Fig. 7.12) . The neurovascular status was intact. Anterior-posterior and lateral radiographs of the foot and ankle were normal. The diagnosis was clearly an acute rupture of the Achilles tendon, and there was no indication for further diagnostic studies.

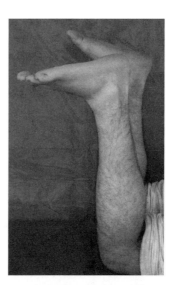

Fig. 7.10. Excess dorsiflexion of the right ankle in a patient suffering from an acute rupture of the Achilles tendon

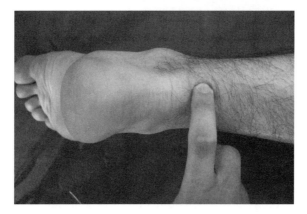

Fig. 7.11. A tender palpable defect was present in the Achilles tendon 4 cm proximal to its insertion (same patient as in Fig. 7.10)

Fig. 7.12. A positive Thompson test for an acute rupture of the Achilles tendon (same patient as in Figs. 7.10 and 7.11)

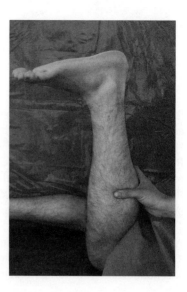

The patient was brought to the operating room and placed prone on the operating table with a tourniquet around his upper thigh. The site of injury, represented by the gap or soft spot, was carefully palpated. The incision was paratendinous and medial, beginning at the soft spot and extending approximately 1.5 cm proximally. The skin and subcutaneous tissue were gently retracted with hooks and the paratenon identified. The sheath was carefully opened, and each edge was tagged with a stay suture. Both stumps of the ruptured tendon were identified and the exact site of rupture carefully noted.

The Achillon was introduced in the closed position under the paratenon in a proximal direction, with the tendon stump held with a small clamp under the instrument. The tendon stump was located between the two internal branches. As the instrument was introduced, it was progressively widened, holding the tendon stump firmly with the clamp. Three sutures were passed from lateral to medial. The instrument was then slowly withdrawn while progressively closing the branches. This maneuver resulted in the sutures sliding from an extracutaneous position to a peritendinous position, and thus the tendon itself was the only tissue held by the sutures. The same sequence was performed on the distal stump with the instrument being introduced under the tendon sheath and pushed until it touched the calcaneum. All the sutures were at this point organized for tightening, which was carried out with corresponding pairs, and the tendon reduction was under direct visual control. The tendon sheath was closed, and then the skin was closed with intradermal sutures. A splint was applied holding the ankle in 30 degrees of flexion prior to moving or waking the patient. Low-molecular-weight heparin (subcutaneous administration) was used for prophylactic anticoagulation for 3 weeks postoperative.

The physical therapist carefully supervised an early functional rehabilitation program, comprised of the four stages discussed above (see Rehabilitation Protocol).

The patient was followed up twice a month. At 3 months he was able to run without pain, and at 5 months he was able to play squash without any symptoms.

Indications and Contraindications

The indication for this technique is an acute (less than 3 weeks) Achilles tendon rupture occurring between 2 and 8 cm above the tuberosity of the calcaneus. Contraindications include the following: chronic rupture greater than 3 weeks in duration, previous local surgery, patients on steroids, open ruptures and lacerations of greater than 6 hours in duration, complex open ruptures with soft tissue defects, and ruptures occurring less than 2 cm below or more than 8 cm above the tuberosity of the calcaneus. More than 90% of ruptures of the Achilles tendon occur in the area between 2 and 8 cm above the calcaneal tuberosity.[16] We believe that ruptures occurring more than 8 cm above the tuberosity (muscular ruptures) can be treated nonoperatively, while ruptures occurring less than 2 cm from the tuberosity necessitate fixation directly to bone.

Discussion

Rupture of the Achilles tendon is a common injury among high-level athletes, recreational sports enthusiasts, and even sedentary individuals. The incidence of ruptures of the Achilles tendon appears to have increased during the past 10 to 15 years.[17] It has been reported that men in the third and fourth decade who play sports occasionally are the typical patients to sustain an acute Achilles tendon rupture.[18,19] Although the diagnosis of a fresh Achilles tendon rupture is relatively straightforward, with both clinical examination and specialized testing available, a number of these injuries are missed at the initial presentation.[20]

Controversy still exists concerning the treatment of a fresh rupture of the Achilles tendon. The original focus was on managing these injuries without surgery with plaster immobilization for a 6- to 8-week period. Initially, many investigators were convinced that the results of nonoperative treatment were equal to those achieved with surgical repair.[21–25] Many of these reports are in the older literature, but there still continue to be reference made to satisfactory results with a nonoperative approach.[1] Other reports focusing on nonoperative management using functional bracing, as opposed to prolonged plaster immobilization, have shown good results.[9,26,27] The major motivating factor for such a nonoperative approach appears to be the wound complication rate with an operative repair.

More recent reports in the literature favor operative treatment of a fresh rupture of the Achilles tendon.[1,12,15] But the exact type of operative procedure and the postoperative regimen remain controversial. Most reports in the literature discuss only one of two possible surgical techniques. The first is an open operative repair with a fairly long incision and possible stripping of the paratenon. The latter should be avoided, if possible, as it provides a valuable blood supply to the damaged tendon. Different techniques of suture repair have been described, and it appears that most surgeons generally favor an end-to-end repair.

The reports in the literature describing a high rate of complications from the formal open approach reflect earlier treatment techniques.[21,23–25] The most frequent complication reported is related to wound healing problems, specifically wound necrosis and infection. It may be related to the longitudinal incision commonly used for the surgical approach, which has been shown to pass through an area of poor vascularity.[28] While there has been a decreasing incidence of wound problems, it remains a definite concern in the operative approach to these injuries. In a retrospective review of 314 patients reflecting open repair between 1980 and 1991, Winter et al.[29] noted nine patients with delayed wound healing, ten with a deep infection requiring further operative treatment, and two patients who developed a sinus necessitating débridement and closure. Cetti et al.[1] reported on open repair in 56 of 111 patients, with a 3.6% incidence of deep wound infection, 2% delayed healing, 10% adhesion of scar, and 12% disturbance of sensibility. Mandelbaum et al.[7] reported two patients developing a superficial wound infection among open repair in 29, responding in both cases to debridement. Soldatis et al.[5] reported on an end-to-end repair in 23 consecutive patients, with two of the 23 patients experiencing delayed wound healing that resolved within 3 months. There were no infections. Bradley and Tibone[6] compared percutaneous versus open repair in a total of 27 patients, 12 of whom underwent a percutaneous repair and 15 an open one. There were no wound problems in either group. We have favored a small longitudinal incision so that we have the ability to extend the approach proximally or distally as the pathology necessitates. Although it has been reported that a transverse incision may result in fewer wound complications,[12,30] such an approach severely restricts the surgeon in gaining additional proximal or distal exposure should the need arise.

Because of the concerns regarding wound healing and infection, a percutaneous approach has been considered as a compromise. The proponents of such a technique favor operative repair of the tendon but have attempted to avoid the soft tissue problems associated with an open repair. Ma and Griffith[13] developed such a technique and reported its application in 18 patients, using small stab incisions along the medial and lateral borders of the tendon and passing sutures through the tendon via these stab incisions. They reported two minor wound complications but no infections, and there were no reruptures. Of 28 patients reported by Rowley and Scotland,[31] 10 were treated with the percutaneous technique, with one patient sustaining an entrapment of the sural nerve. The authors concluded that the operative repair group was more likely to recover nearly normal plantarflexion strength, and the patients returned to activity sooner than the nonoperatively treated group.

Other authors have had less favorable results after the percutaneous repair, with major complications involving sural nerve entrapment. Klein et al.[32] reported on 38 patients with a 38% incidence of nerve entrapment, including the necessity for a second operative procedure to remove the offending suture and free the nerve. Nerve entrapment has also been reported by Rowley and Scotland,[31] Steele et al.,[33] and Aracil et al.[34] FitzGibbons et al.[35] reported on two sural nerve injuries, one complete, among 14 patients. Buchgraber and Pässler[36] reported on 59 patients treated with a percutaneous technique. The patients were divided into two groups, one undergoing functional rehabilitation and the other cast immobilization. The authors noted sensory impairment in the territory of the sural nerve in almost one quarter of their 59 patients treated with a percutaneous technique. Although a major reason behind the percutaneous technique is its lower incidence of wound problems, the same authors noted delayed wound healing problems with two patients in each group. Using fresh-frozen below-knee cadaver specimens, Hockenbury and Johns[37] compared in vitro percutaneous repair versus open repair of the Achilles tendon following a transverse tenotomy. One group had an open repair using the Bunnell suture technique, while the other had percutaneous repair using the technique of Ma and Griffith. The tendons repaired with the open technique showed greater resistance to separation of the repair site with increasing ankle dorsiflexion, as compared to the percutaneous group (a 10-mm gap occurred with a mean of 27.6 degrees of ankle dorsiflexion in the open group, and at a mean of 14.1 degrees in the percutaneous group; $p < .05$). In addition, using the percutaneous technique, the tendon stumps were malaligned in four of five specimens. Even more significant, the authors demonstrated entrapment of the sural nerve in three of five specimens using the percutaneous technique. They concluded that percutaneous repair of a ruptured Achilles tendon provides approximately 50% of the initial strength afforded by open repair and places the sural nerve at risk for injury.

A report by Sutherland and Maffulli[38] reported on 31 patients undergoing repair of an acute rupture through a modified percutaneous technique. There were five sural nerve injuries (16%), three of which resolved in 6 to 9 months. One patient with persistent symptoms refused further intervention. The other patient underwent exploration; the findings revealed the sural nerve to be transfixed by a suture. This patient's symptoms resolved 3 months after the second intervention. In a recent study of 124 patients treated with a different instrument (Tenolig®, FH Orthopedics, Quimper, France) for a percutaneous repair, the authors noted eight sural nerve injuries, 10% rerupture, and 10 patients with skin necrosis.[39] Two studies in the current literature comparing percutaneous versus open repair have favored the percutaneous method because of a lower incidence of wound problems.[10,11] But there was still an incidence of sural nerve disturbance in both percutaneous groups of 4.5% to 10.5%. And even a formal open repair does not ensure that the sural nerve will escape injury, as noted in a retrospective review by Winter et al.,[29] in which there were four sural nerve injuries among 314 patients treated between 1980 and 1991 with a formal open repair. Based on our cadaver study, it was clear that this procedure could be performed without entrapping the sural nerve in the suture loop. While reports of sural nerve injury still exist in the literature, following open and particularly percutaneous techniques, our clinical results have shown no neurologic disturbance in any of our patients, and thus no sural nerve injury to date.

The problem of rerupture exists among patients treated nonoperatively as well as with any type of surgical procedure. In most reported series, some type of protection (cast or brace) has been utilized for approximately 3 months, and rerupture usually occurs within 2 to 3 months following removal of the protective device. However, there is another cause of failure of the repair, and this is related to patient compliance. Certainly, no tendon will be sufficiently healed and strong enough to withstand normal loading during the first 6 to 8 weeks. Therefore, if a patient removes the protective device during this period, the so-called rerupture is simply the repair coming apart *before* it heals. Most studies have shown a higher incidence of rerupture in those patients treated with a percutaneous procedure. In the study by Bradley and Tibone,[6] there were two reruptures in the group of 12 treated with the percutaneous technique, and none in the open repair group of patients who had a gastroc-soleus fascial graft. The authors noted a more symmetrical tendon size in the percutaneous group. Their recommendation was for a percutaneous repair in the recreational athlete and in patients concerned with cosmesis, and an open repair for all high-caliber athletes "who cannot afford any chance of rerupture." In the study by Sutherland and Maffulli,[38] there were two reruptures among 31 patients with a modified percutaneous technique, at 11 and 15 months postoperative. Aracil et al.[34] reported on two ruptures among six patients who underwent Achilles tendon repair with the original percutaneous technique of Ma and Griffith. They surmised that this "blind" technique may result in inadequate opposition of the tendon ends. In the previously cited study by Maes et al.,[39] there was a 10% incidence of rerupture with their percutaneous technique. But other reports demonstrate more reruptures in patients treated with an open technique versus percutaneous, but they are in the minority.

There has been a more recent interest in avoiding prolonged immobilization following both nonoperative and operative treatment. McComis et al.[26] used functional bracing for the nonoperative treatment of 15 patients with acute Achilles tendon rupture. The goals of such treatment, as outlined by the authors, were to prevent the musculoskeletal changes associated with immobilization, to reduce the time needed for rehabilitation, and to facilitate an early return to work and preinjury activities. They assessed functional performance in these patients (walking, rising on the toes, and hopping) in comparison to the uninjured extremities of an age- and gender-matched group of controls. With the exception of increased dorsiflexion of the ankle in the study group, they failed to detect any significant differences between the groups in the clinical and functional parameters assessed.

Mortensen et al.[4] reported on a prospective study of 71 patients who underwent an open repair, with one group assigned to cast immobilization and non–weight bearing for 8 weeks, and the other to a removable brace with early restricted motion and partial weight bearing beginning after the fourth week. The authors noted that early restricted motion shortened the time needed for rehabilitation, but unloaded exercises did not prevent muscle atrophy. Carter et al.[9] treated 21 patients with surgical repair and used a functional orthosis postoperatively. These patients were only allowed toe-touch weight bearing for the first 6 to 8 weeks but allowed unrestricted ankle plantarflexion and dorsiflexion to neutral. Sixteen patients returned to their preinjury level of activity, and only one was unsatisfied with the end result. Compared to the contralateral limb, dorsiflexion was increased an average of only 2 degrees and plantarflexion was unchanged. Strength, power, and endurance were similar between the injured and uninjured extremity.

Sölveborn and Moberg[8] prospectively studied 17 patients who were allowed immediate free ankle motion after surgical repair. Weight bearing in a special orthosis was also possible, and no organized rehabilitation program was instituted. There were no reruptures, and at 1-year follow-up there were 15 excellent and two good results according to their scoring system. Six patients were noted to have excellent results as early as 3 months postoperative. Buchgraber and Pässler[36] assigned their 48 patients to two different groups after all underwent percutaneous repair of their Achilles tendon rupture. Thirty patients were selected for functional postoperative treatment consisting of pain-limited weight bearing in a special shoe as well as range of motion and isometric exercises. The remaining patients were immobilized in equinus for 2 weeks and placed in a weight- bearing cast for 4 weeks. Although the authors noted problems with wound healing and sural nerve injury in both groups (as we previously commented), the functional group required significantly less sick leave time and reported a significantly higher visual analogue scale rating as to the subjectively perceived outcome of surgery. For this reason, we use an early functional rehabilitation program with early partial weight bearing and early ankle and foot range-of-motion exercises.

Kakiuchi[14] described in 1995 his combined open and percutaneous procedure, using only a limited incision at the site of rupture, and introducing sutures in a percutaneous fashion proximal and distal to the rupture site. He divided 34 patients with acute Achilles tendon ruptures into two groups. One group of 14 underwent a standard open repair, while the other 20 patients were treated with his new combined procedure. He had only 22 patients available for follow-up, 12 in the combined procedure group and 10 who had the open repair. His results showed the patients in the combined group had significantly better relief of symptoms during everyday activities, better single-limb hopping, and a greater chance to return to sports. He also found a better cosmetic result with the combined procedure. One patient treated with the combined procedure had an increase in ankle dorsiflexion, representing lengthening of the tendon. Kakiuchi attributed this to probable passing of the sutures through injured parts of the tendon. Also with his new procedure there was one case of transient impairment of sural nerve function, which may have been due to repeated piercing of the skin by the needle in search of the suture guide. In his article, Kakiuchi states that passing sutures through the skin, intact tendon, and holes in the suture guide is a "blind" part of the procedure that "requires the surgeon to direct the needle repeatedly against the suture guide." This new procedure of Kakiuchi was the impetus for me to develop a new surgical technique with a new instrument in order to combine the advantages of the open and percutaneous approaches. With the Achillon system, and through a limited incision at the actual site of rupture, we are able to introduce sutures in a percutaneous fashion proximal and distal to the rupture site. This allows for direct visualization of the repair site, providing precise opposition of the tendon ends and restoring accurate tension in the muscle-tendon unit, while limiting the surgical dissection and disturbance of local blood supply. The postoperative program provides early weight bearing and ankle range of motion, and our results justify continued use of this technique. Three recent reports using the exact surgical technique and Achillon instrument that I developed provide further confirmation of its important role in repair of acute Achilles tendon ruptures.[12,40,41]

References

1. Cetti R, Christensen SE, Ejsted R, et al. Operative versus nonoperative treatment of Achilles tendon rupture. A prospective randomized study and review of the literature. Am J Sports Med 1993;21:791–9.
2. Leppilahti J, Orava S. Total Achilles tendon rupture. A review. Sports Med 1998;25: 79–100.
3. Maffulli N. Rupture of the Achilles tendon. J Bone Joint Surg [Am] 1999;81:1019–36.
4. Mortensen HM, Skov O, Jensen PE. Early motion of the ankle after operative treatment of a rupture of the Achilles tendon. A prospective, randomized clinical and radiographic study. J Bone Joint Surg [Am] 1999;81:983–90.
5. Soldatis JJ, Goodfellow DB, Wilber JH. End-to-end operative repair of Achilles tendon rupture. Am J Sports Med 1997;25:90–5.

6. Bradley JP, Tibone JE. Percutaneous and open surgical repairs of Achilles tendon ruptures. A comparative study. Am J Sports Med 1990;18:188–95.
7. Mandelbaum BR, Myerson MS, Forster R. Achilles tendon ruptures. A new method of repair, early range of motion, and functional rehabilitation. Am J Sports Med 1995;23:392–5.
8. Solveborn SA, Moberg A. Immediate free ankle motion after surgical repair of acute Achilles tendon ruptures. Am J Sports Med 1994;22:607–10.
9. Carter TR, Fowler PJ, Blokker C. Functional postoperative treatment of Achilles tendon repair. Am J Sports Med 1992;20:459–62.
10. Haji A, Sahai A, Symes A, Vyas JK. Percutaneous versus open tendo achillis repair. Foot Ankle Int 2004;25:215–8.
11. Cretnik A, Kosanovic M, Smrkolj V. Percutaneous versus open repair of the ruptured Achilles tendon: a comparative study. Am J Sports Med 2005;33:1369–79.
12. Calder JD, Saxby TS. Independent evaluation of a recently described Achilles tendon repair technique. Foot Ankle Int 2006;27:93–6.
13. Ma GW, Griffith TG. Percutaneous repair of acute closed ruptured Achilles tendon: a new technique. Clin Orthop 1977;247–55.
14. Kakiuchi M. A combined open and percutaneous technique for repair of tendo Achillis. Comparison with open repair. J Bone Joint Surg [Br] 1995;77:60–3.
15. Assal M, Jung M, Stern R, et al. Limited open repair of Achilles tendon ruptures: a technique with a new instrument and findings of a prospective multicenter study. J Bone Joint Surg [Am] 2002;84A:161–70.
16. DiStefano VJ, Nixon JE. Achilles tendon rupture: pathogenesis, diagnosis, and treatment by a modified pullout wire technique. J Trauma 1972;12:671–7.
17. Leppilahti J, Puranen J, Orava S. Incidence of Achilles tendon rupture. Acta Orthop Scand 1996;67:277–9.
18. Boyden EM, Kitaoka HB, Cahalan TD, et al. Late versus early repair of Achilles tendon rupture. Clinical and biomechanical evaluation. Clin Orthop 1995;150–8.
19. Hattrup SJ, Johnson KA. A review of ruptures of the Achilles tendon. Foot Ankle 1985;6:34–8.
20. Inglis AE, Scott WN, Sculco TP, et al. Ruptures of the tendo achillis. An objective assessment of surgical and non-surgical treatment. J Bone Joint Surg [Am] 1976;58:990–3.
21. Carden DG, Noble J, Chalmers J, et al. Rupture of the calcaneal tendon. The early and late management. J Bone Joint Surg [Br] 1987;69:416–20.
22. Gillies H, Chalmers J. The management of fresh ruptures of the tendo achillis. J Bone Joint Surg [Am] 1970;52:337–43.
23. Lea RB, Smith L. Non-surgical treatment of tendo achillis rupture. J Bone Joint Surg [Am] 1972;54:1398–407.
24. Nistor L. Surgical and non-surgical treatment of Achilles Tendon rupture. A prospective randomized study. J Bone Joint Surg [Am] 1981;63:394–9.
25. Stein SR, Luekens CA Jr. Closed treatment of Achilles tendon ruptures. Orthop Clin North Am 1976;7:241–6.
26. McComis GP, Nawoczenski DA, DeHaven KE. Functional bracing for rupture of the Achilles tendon. Clinical results and analysis of ground-reaction forces and temporal data. J Bone Joint Surg [Am] 1997;79:1799–808.
27. Thermann H, Zwipp H, Tscherne H. [Functional treatment concept of acute rupture of the Achilles tendon. 2 years results of a prospective randomized study]. Unfallchirurg 1995;98:21–32.
28. Haertsch PA. The blood supply to the skin of the leg: a post-mortem investigation. Br J Plast Surg 1981;34:470–77.
29. Winter E, Weisc K, Weller S, et al. Surgical repair of Achilles tendon rupture. Comparison of surgical with conservative treatment. Arch Orthop Trauma Surg 1998;117:364–7.

30. Aldam CH. Repair of calcaneal tendon ruptures. A safe technique. J Bone Joint Surg [Br] 1989;71:486–8.
31. Rowley DI, Scotland TR. Rupture of the Achilles tendon treated by a simple operative procedure. Injury 1982;14:252–4.
32. Klein W, Lang DM, Saleh M. The use of the Ma-Griffith technique for percutaneous repair of fresh ruptured tendo Achillis. Chir Organi Mov 1991;76:223–8.
33. Steele G, Harter R, Ting A. Comparison of functional ability following percutaneous and open surgical repairs of acutely ruptured Achilles tendons. J Sport Rehabil 1993;2:115–27.
34. Aracil J, Pina A, Lozano JA, et al. Percutaneous suture of Achilles tendon ruptures. Foot Ankle 1992;13:350–1.
35. FitzGibbons RE, Hefferon J, Hill J. Percutaneous Achilles tendon repair [see comments]. Am J Sports Med 1993;21:724–7.
36. Buchgraber A, Passler HH. Percutaneous repair of Achilles tendon rupture. Immobilization versus functional postoperative treatment. Clin Orthop 1997;113–22.
37. Hockenbury RT, Johns JC. A biomechanical in vitro comparison of open versus percutaneous repair of tendon Achilles. Foot Ankle 1990;11:67–72.
38. Sutherland A, Maffulli N. A modified technique of percutaneous repair of ruptured Achilles tendon. Oper Orthop Traumat 1999;7:288–95.
39. Maes R, Copin G, Averous C. Is percutaneous repair of the Achilles tendon a safe technique? A study of 124 cases. Acta Orthop Belg 2006;72:179–83.
40. Marsh J, CS. Ankle fractures. In: Bucholz R, Heckman J, Court-Brown C, eds. Rockwood and Green's Fractures in Adults, 6th ed. Philadelphia: Lippincott Williams & Wilkins, 2006:2238–41.
41. Rippstein P, Easley M. "Mini-open" repair for acute Achilles tendon ruptures. Tech Foot Ankle Surg 2006;5:3–8.

8

Formal Open Repair of the Achilles Tendon

Claude T. Moorman III and Maria K.A. Kaseta

Acute ruptures of the Achilles tendon are common injuries associated with trauma, male gender, obesity, and a history of injected corticosteroids.[1] Although there is a significant increase in the incidence of Achilles tendon injuries over the last two decades,[2] there is no consensus regarding the optimal management (operative vs. nonoperative) of acute ruptures of the Achilles tendon.[3–7] This chapter describes the operative technique favored by the senior author as well as a physical therapy protocol that has resulted in excellent outcomes.

A number of studies have shown that surgical repair results in less morbidity and improved function. For example, surgically repaired tendons are at lower risk of rerupture,[4,7,8] and patients who elect surgery achieve normal push-off power.[9,10] One randomized prospective study compared operative versus nonoperative treatment of acute ruptures of the Achilles tendon in 111 patients and demonstrated better results (resuming sports activities, fewer subjective complaints) in the operative group at 1 year follow-up, although there were fewer minor complications in the nonoperative group.[11] Other advantages of surgical repair include decreased ankle stiffness and calf atrophy, fewer tendo-cutaneous adhesions, and a lower risk of thrombophlebitis.[12,13]

Open operative treatment of acute ruptures of the Achilles tendon is probably the method of choice for athletes and patients who wish to continue with high-demand physical activity.[4,9] Two recent meta-analyses of randomized controlled trials showed that operative management has a reduced risk of rerupture compared with conservative measures, but was associated with an increased risk of complications including wound infections, delayed wound healing, adhesions, and disturbed sensations.[4,7]

Case Study

While playing golf, a 35-year-old man ran up a hill, felt a sudden onset of pain behind his right ankle, and heard a popping sound. He turned around, as he thought he had been struck with an errant golf ball. He came to the clinic 6 days later with right lower extremity pain (2 on a 10-point visual analogue scale). His aching pain was continuous, was worse in the morning,

J.A. Nunley (ed.), *The Achilles Tendon: Treatment and Rehabilitation*,
DOI: 10.1007/978-1-387-79206-4_8, © Springer Science+Business Media, LLC 2009

and aggravated when standing. He had been treating his pain with ice and non–weight bearing (by sitting and lying down).

On physical examination, the patient was healthy except for non–weight bearing on the right side. His right ankle range of motion was 30 degrees of dorsiflexion, 0 degrees of plantarflexion, 15 degrees of inversion, and 30 degrees of eversion. The Thompson test was positive, and a mild ankle effusion was noted. His knee and hindfoot were in neutral alignment. He had a palpable defect in his Achilles tendon 3 cm proximal to the calcaneal insertion with tenderness at this site. His plantarflexion strength was 3/5. No additional motor or sensory deficits were noted. His peripheral pulses were normal with no edema. His personal and family histories were unremarkable. The clinical diagnosis was that he had a right Achilles tendon rupture.

The operation was performed 2 days after his initial clinical examination. Preoperative regional anesthesia was induced in the anesthesia holding area. The patient was taken to the operating room and placed in the prone position. The lower extremity was scrubbed using Hibiclens and alcohol, prepped using DuraPrep, and then draped using sterile drapes and towels. The extremity was exsanguinated using an Esmarch and the tourniquet was inflated to 300 mm Hg. The tourniquet time for the procedure was 45 minutes.

An incision was made along the lateral portion of the midline. Dissection was carried down to identify the sural nerve that was retracted carefully. The peritenon was then identified and incised longitudinally over the torn portion. Both ends of the tear were then delivered into the wound site. Tajima sutures with No. 2 Orthocord suture were placed into position using tapered needles. Two Tajima stitches were placed proximally and two were placed distally. The foot was held in a 90-degree neutral position and the sutures were tied down securely. Next, interrupted 0 Vicryl sutures were used to repair the tendon edges over the scaffolding, then the paratenon was closed with 2-0 Vicryl over the site. The subcutaneous tissue was closed using 2-0 Vicryl. A running 3-0 Prolene subcuticular stitch was used for the skin. A bulky dry sterile dressing and a posterior splint were applied.

There was minimal blood loss, no drains, and no complications.

After the procedure, the patient was placed in a posterior splint and was non–weight bearing for 10 days.

At 10 days, the splint was removed and he was placed in a Cam walker with the ankle in a neutral position for weight bearing. During this period, the patient began 30 cycles of rebound active dorsiflexion, three times per day, to provide gentle stress to the healing collagen to encourage healing along the lines of stress.

At 6 weeks, the patient was given the option of using an ankle-foot orthosis in his regular shoe, but could return to the boot as needed. Thus, the injury was protected with non–weight bearing and a boot or an ankle-foot orthosis for 3 months after the operation.

At 3 months, weight bearing as tolerated was permitted in the absence of any immobilization. He was permitted to begin progression back to his sport, but not allowed full participation until 6 months. The patient was evaluated clinically and subjectively. He went back to his athletic activities after 6 months and on last follow-up had a normal tendon contour, full range of motion, and full strength with resumption of all activities.

In the attempt to improve the overall outcome of patients with Achilles tendon rupture and to reduce complications, a number of different surgical techniques have been described including open,[14,15] percutaneous,[16,17] and combined procedures.[18] Open surgical methods are of two types: those involving direct tendon repair with different suture techniques (e.g., Kessler, Bunnel, Tajima, Krakow, triple bundle),[19] and those involving reconstruction using grafts (e.g., gastrocnemius fascia, plantaris tendon, fascia lata, peroneus brevis, flexor digitorum longus [FDL], flexor hallucis longus [FHL]),[9] or synthetic materials (e.g., carbon fiber, Dacron grafts).[20,21]

The choice of surgical procedure requires consideration of a number of factors including mechanism of injury; the time from the initial injury[3,5,10,15,19,22]; the presence of connective tissue diseases (which usually requires augmentation)[10]; local factors (e.g., ischemia, atrophy of gastrocnemius-soleus muscle, scars, infections)[5,10]; and demographics such as age, gender, and athletic activity of the patient.[10] According to Wapner,[10] primary end-to-end repair can be done up to 3 months postoperatively. In general, however, the longer the time from the initial injury, the less likely a primary end-to-end repair can be performed successfully with acceptable physician and patient outcomes.

Several authors define chronic ruptures of the Achilles tendon as injuries left untreated for more than 4 weeks.[3] The gap between ruptured ends, assessed preoperatively with MRI and intraoperatively after excision of the impaired tissue, is the determining factor for the type of surgical repair. In a neg lected Achilles tendon rupture, the subsequent contraction of the tendon and the formation of fibrous scar tissue make even relatively small gaps less likely to achieve a successful end-to-end repair.[5,22] An end-to-end anastomosis is usually possible in 1- to 2-cm defects.[5,22] For 2- to 5-cm defects, either V-Y myotendinous lengthening, graft augmentation, or both are surgical options.[5,22] For defects larger than 5 cm, a graft reconstruction method should be employed.[5] An FHL transfer seems to be a reliable and effective way to deal with large, chronic defects.[5,6,10]

If surgical repair is chosen, it is recommended to wait for 4 to 7 days, to allow for the reduction of swelling and to lessen the degree of fraying and friability of the tendon that could occur if the repair is performed immediately postinjury.[4,23,24] We prefer to perform the repair within 2 weeks of the injury to minimize gapping and to facilitate tissue handling. As always, the optimal management plan should include not only the selection of the surgical technique but also the patient's health status, expectations, and goals.

Primary Repair Using the Tajima Suture Technique

We favor the (four-strand) Tajima suture technique, which is widely used by hand surgeons for flexor tendon repair and is an excellent soft tissue–holding suture.[25,26] The patient is positioned prone with the feet lying just over the end of the table. Using a thigh tourniquet is optional, but advisable. The contralateral extremity is draped so it can be used for intraoperative comparison of resting dynamic tension of the repaired tendon.[5,9]

A linear posterolateral incision, approximately 10 cm long, is made about 1 cm lateral to the tendon (Fig. 8.1). The incision ends proximal to where the shoe counter strikes the heel. It has to be off-center to prevent later irritation by shoes, which can happen if the incision is directly over the tendon midline.[19] Care should be taken to maintain full thickness and to avoid undermining the skin flaps. The sural nerve is usually found directly under the incision and must be carefully protected. The incision is deepened sharply into the deep fascia. Finally, the deep fascia and the peritendinous tissues are incised longitudinally to expose the rupture. The incision should be made through all three layers (deep fascia, mesotenon, thin layer closest to the tendon) directly to the middle of the tendon itself.[23] Gently retract the skin throughout the procedure using only skin hooks or hand-held retractors.[23]

The hematoma is evacuated, and the quality and extent of damage are assessed. Any obvious redundant, detached, or devitalized tissue should be sharply excised.[3,19,23] Posteriorly, the tendon is invariably separated while anteriorly it is possible to find some fibers intact, but attenuated.[23]

Two sutures are used on each side of the rupture and are tied in the middle (Fig. 8.2). A long, tapered needle is used with nonabsorbable No. 5 polyester suture material. The needle is passed through one of the ruptured ends of the tendon and then out of the tendon 5 cm proximal to or distal from the injured end. This suture then is passed across and exits the tendon. Next the suture is passed back down within the tendon and out of the injured surface. The process is repeated for the opposite side of the tendon. The knots are tied within the tendon to unite the injured ends. This process is repeated, only this time the suture exits the tendon 2.5 cm from the cut surfaces (Fig. 8.2).

A most important aspect of surgical repair is correct tensioning of the tendon. The ankle is held in neutral position as sutures are tied. Each strand is pulled to obtain a sense of the correct tension and compared to the opposite limb.[5] Often the tendon fibers will not be in continuity. The proximal and distal ends of the tendon are "milked" together along the tensioned sutures to the point of contact, for a scaffold of healing. Simple 0-braided absorbable sutures are used to further approximate the repair (Fig. 8.3).

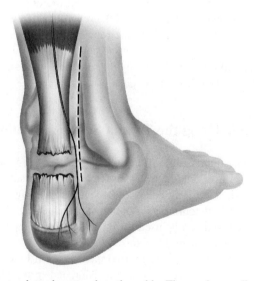

Fig. 8.1. The posterolateral approach to the ankle. The sural nerve lies underneath the incision plane, so it must be carefully identified and protected

The peritenon is a major source of blood supply to the tendon as well as the border between the tendon and the subcutaneous layer preventing adhesions. This layer is closed carefully using 2-0 absorbable suture (Fig. 8.4).[5] The subcutaneous layer is closed with interrupted 2-0 braided absorbable sutures. The skin is closed with a running 3-0 monofilament nonabsorbable pullout suture. Swelling of the repaired tendon may complicate wound closure, and a fasciotomy of the posterior aspect of the leg has been proposed to resolve this issue.[5] The neurovascular status of the limb must be assessed. A posterior ankle splint set in a neutral position is applied, and the operated limb is elevated on a frame. The sutures are removed about 2 weeks postsurgery.

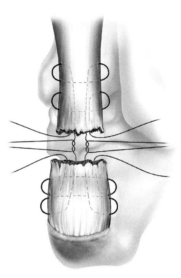

Fig. 8.2. The Tajima suture with four strands. Note that one set of sutures exits the tissue at 5 cm, and a parallel set of sutures exits the tissue at 2.5 cm

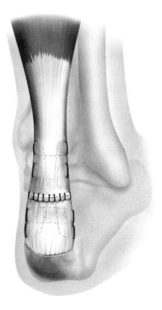

Fig. 8.3. Tendon ends approximated further with interrupted suture

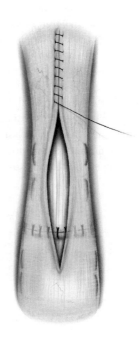

Fig. 8.4. Retinacular layer closure

Rehabilitation

Physical therapy is an essential component to improve the patient's postinjury recovery of activity and satisfaction.[27,28] An early start to rehabilitation is recommended as there is a significant decrease in complication rates in patients treated with surgery and early mobilization versus those treated with surgery and immobilization.[4,7] Prolonged immobilization is associated with an increased incidence of calf atrophy, articular cartilage weakening and degeneration, osteoporosis, skin necrosis, adhesions, deep venous thrombosis, and even pulmonary embolism.[3,22] A meta-analysis confirms that there are more excellent subjective responses, fewer scar adhesions, and fewer transient sural nerve deficits in patients who began an early rehabilitation protocol (when there was no difference in rerupture rate and percentage of superficial and deep infections among them).[29]

The posterior splint is removed within 10 to 14 days during which weight bearing is forbidden. When the splint is removed, a walking boot (neutral position) is applied and patients start progressively weight bearing as they feel comfortable. Patients are encouraged to perform mobilization of the involved ankle three times per day by performing 30 cycles of active dorsiflexion-recoil passive plantarflexion with the knee flexed 90 degrees (Fig. 8.5A,B). No active plantarflexion is permitted (Fig. 8.5C). Active dorsiflexion is used to provide gentle traction to the repair to promote collagen healing along lines of stress.[13] Recoil plantarflexion (not active) allows a return to neutral position. After 6 weeks the patient can switch to an ankle-foot orthosis or remain in a boot (usually 50% each). At 3 months the patient is weight bearing without immobilization. Generally, 6 months are required for a full return to sports.

Over the past 5 years, the senior author has performed this surgical technique on more than 100 acute Achilles tendon ruptures. Despite the proximity of this approach to the sural nerve, no sural nerve palsies occurred. Complications

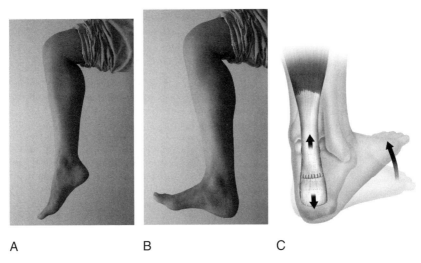

Fig. 8.5. (A,B) Active dorsiflexion-recoil passive plantarflexion with the knee flexed 90 degrees; 30 cycles three times per day. (C) No active plantarflexion

were few, as only four patients had delayed wound healing. There were no infections or other major complications. There was only one rerupture in a weight lifter, who, against medical advice, decided to return to full activity 3 months postoperatively. All but one patient returned to their full levels of previous activity.

Other Surgical Options

Watson et al.[30] tested three suture methods (the Kessler, the Bunnell, and the Krackow locking loop) as to the initial strength of Achilles tendon repair. The locking loop suture method was significantly stronger than either of the other two configurations. The latter two did not differ significantly from each other.

Jaakkola and colleagues[31] compared the tensile strength of ruptured Achilles tendons repaired using either the triple-bundle technique or the Krakow locking loop technique. They showed a significantly stronger repair with the triple-bundle technique. Jaakkola et al.[32] evaluated the triple-bundle technique for acute Achilles tendon rupture repair followed by early post-operative ankle range of motion versus nonoperative treatment with delayed ankle range of motion in 73 patients. They found operative treatment reduced immobilization and weight-bearing time. Yet, at a follow-up of 3.5 years or greater, there was no statistical difference in American Orthopaedic Foot and Ankle Society [AOFAS] hindfoot scores, strength, or patient satisfaction between the two groups. There were more complications in the nonoperative group with three reruptures (7.7%) versus only one deep wound dehiscence in the operative group (3%).

Mandelbaum and coworkers[12] used a Krackow suture technique[33] and early postoperative mobilization in 32 patients, achieving excellent results and no reruptures. All patients returned to preinjury activity levels at an average of 4 months after repair. By 12 months, there were no significant differences in ankle motion, isokinetic strength, or endurance compared with the uninvolved side.

Maffulli et al.[34] used a single modified Kessler suture in two groups. The first group followed an early weight-bearing ankle mobilization protocol, while the second group followed a more traditional postoperative protocol. Both groups had a similar fraction of excellent results and no reruptures, but the first group had faster recovery and return to work with less use of rehabilitation recourses. Gastroc-soleus muscle strength deficit and muscle atrophy, however, were not prevented.

Finally, Speck and Klaue[13] used a Kessler-type suture and simple apposition sutures combined with an accelerated rehabilitation protocol in 20 patients with excellent results and no reruptures. All patients reached their preinjury levels of sports activities with no significant difference in ankle mobility or isokinetic strength.

Potential Complications

There are several possible complications of Achilles tendon injuries. One large review reported the complication rate in operatively treated patients was 20%, but most complications were minor.[35] Skin complications include keloid formation, wound necrosis, and skin and soft tissue defects, any of which could require free tissue transfers.[9,36] Adhesions of the tendon to overlying skin are considered minor complications and usually require little, if any, treatment. In a few cases, surgical lysis and early mobilization are recommended.[23]

After an open repair, the tendon can thicken by up to three to four times its natural size[34]; however, this usually resolves within 18 months.

Ankle stiffness is a result of failure to achieve sufficient tendon length during the procedure and subsequent prolonged immobilization. Excessive tendon length is also unacceptable because push-off strength would be inadequate.[5] If normal strength has not completely been restored after 6 months, the patient must continue rehabilitation, because improvement is expected to continue.[9] Oral or intravenous antibiotics treat infections, but surgical debridement may also be necessary.[23]

Reruptures can usually be controlled by closely following the postoperative rehabilitation protocol.[7] In the unfortunate case of a rerupture, the patient should be managed as though he or she has an acute rupture. It might be a good idea to reconstruct the tendon with an FHL transfer because rerupture has not been reported with that technique.[10] Sural nerve damage and sural neuroma usually occur after a lateral approach; however, we still prefer a lateral approach because, with careful incision and identification of the nerve, this complication easily can be avoided. Our experience with this approach is that the incidence of wound healing problems is very small.[37] It is important to leave the surrounding tissue as a protective layer after identification of the nerve. In the case of sural neuroma formation, it has been proposed to transect the nerve more proximally where the subcutaneous tissue is intact.[10]

Achilles tendon rupture is a condition that responds well to surgical repair. The technique described is a relatively simple, robust repair with a relatively few, minor wound complications. The immediate positioning of the ankle postoperatively in neutral position with an early mobilization rehabilitation protocol is important for a successful outcome.

References

1. Seeger JD, West WA, Fife D, Noel GJ, Johnson LN, Walker AM. Achilles tendon rupture and its association with fluoroquinolone antibiotics and other potential risk factors in a managed care population. Pharmacoepidemiol Drug Saf 2006;15(11):784–92.
2. Maffulli N, Waterston SW, Squair J, et al. Changing incidence of Achilles tendon rupture in Scotland: a 15-year study. Clin J Sport Med 1999;9(3):157–60.
3 Tafuri SA, Daly N. Achilles tendon trauma. In: Banks AS, et al., eds. McGlamry's Comprehensive Textbook of Foot and Ankle Surgery, 3rd ed., Philadelphia, Lippincott Williams & Wilkins. 2006;1706–23.
4. Wong J, Barrass V, Maffulli N. Quantitative review of operative and nonoperative management of Achilles tendon ruptures. Am J Sports Med 2002;30(4):565–75.
5. Myerson MS. Achilles tendon ruptures. AAOS Instructional Course Lectures 1999;48:219–30.
6. Wapner KL. Achilles tendon ruptures and posterior heel pain. In: Kelikian AS, ed. Operative Treatment of the Foot and Ankle. Stamford, Connecticut. APPLETON & LANGE. 1999:369–87.
7. Khan RJ, Fick D, Keogh A, et al. Treatment of acute Achilles tendon ruptures. A meta-analysis of randomized, controlled trials. J Bone Joint Surg [Am] 2005;87(10):2202–10.
8 Bhandari M, Guyatt GH, Siddiqui F, et al. Treatment of acute Achilles tendon ruptures: a systematic overview and metaanalysis. Clin Orthop Rel Res 2002;(400):190–200.
9. Coughlin MJ. Disorders of tendons. In: Coughlin MJ, Mann RA, eds. Surgery of the Foot and Ankle, 7th ed., St Louis, Missouri. Mosby, Inc. 1999:786–861.
10. Wapner KL. Chronic Achilles tendon rupture. In: Nunley JA, Pfeffer GB, Sanders RW, Trepman E, eds. Advanced Reconstruction Foot and Ankle. American Academy of Orthopedic Surgery, Rosemont. 2004: 163–8.
11. Cetti R, Christensen SE, Ejsted R, et al. Operative versus nonoperative treatment of Achilles tendon rupture. A prospective randomized study and review of the literature. Am J Sports Med 1993;21(6):791–9.
12. Mandelbaum BR, Myerson MS, Forster R. Achilles tendon ruptures. A new method of repair, early range of motion, and functional rehabilitation. Am J Sports Med 1995;23(4):392–5.
13. Speck M, Klaue K. Early full weightbearing and functional treatment after surgical repair of acute Achilles tendon rupture. Am J Sports Med 1998;26(6):789–93.
14. Assal M, Jung M, Stern R, et al. Limited open repair of Achilles tendon ruptures: a technique with a new instrument and findings of a prospective multicenter study. J Bone Joint Surg [Am] 2002;84–A(2):161–70.
15. Lennox DW, Wang GJ, McCue FC, et al. The operative treatment of Achilles tendon injuries. Clin Orthop Rel Res 1980;(148):152–5.
16. Ma GW, Griffith TG. Percutaneous repair of acute closed ruptured Achilles tendon: a new technique. Clin Orthop Rel Res 1977;(128):247–55.
17. Zandbergen RA, de Boer SF, Swierstra BA, et al. Surgical treatment of Achilles tendon rupture: examination of strength of 3 types of suture techniques in a cadaver model. Acta Orthop 2005;76(3):408–11.
18. Kakiuchi M. A combined open and percutaneous technique for repair of tendo Achillis. Comparison with open repair. J Bone Joint Surg [Br] 1995;77(1):60–3.
19. Azar FM, Pickering RM. Traumatic Disorders. In: Canale T, ed. Campbell's Operative Orthopaedics, 9th ed., St Louis, Missouri. Mosby-Year Book, Inc. 1998:1405–49.
20. Levy M, Velkes S, Goldstein J, et al. A method of repair for Achilles tendon ruptures without cast immobilization. Preliminary report. Clin Orthop Rel Res 1984;(187):199–204.
21. Jenkins DH, Forster IW, McKibbin B, et al. Induction of tendon and ligament formation by carbon implants. J Bone Joint Surg [Br] 1977;59–B(1):53–7.

22. Canete AC, Deiparine HP. Treatment of chronic Achilles tendon rupture with triple bundle suturing technique and early rehabilitation: early results. Tech Orthop 2006;21(2):134–42.

23. Schuberth JM. Achilles tendon trauma. In: Scurran BL, ed. Foot and Ankle Trauma, 2nd ed., New York, NY. Churchill Livingstone Inc. 1996:205–31.

24. Miller MD, Howard RF, Plancher KD. Achilles tendon Repair. In: Lampert R, ed. Surgical Atlas of Sports Medicine. Printed in Hong Kong. Saunders. An imprint of Elsevier Science (USA). 2003:183–6.

25. Urbaniak JR. Repair of the flexor pollicis longus. Hand Clin 1985;1(1):69–76.

26. Tran HN, Cannon DL, Lieber RL, et al. In vitro cyclic tensile testing of combined peripheral and core flexor tenorrhaphy suture techniques. J Hand Surg [Am] 2002;27(3):518–24.

27. Rajasekar K, Gholve P, Faraj AA, et al. A subjective outcome analysis of tendo-Achilles rupture. J Foot Ankle Surg 2005;44(1):32–36.

28. Dugan DH, Hobler CK. Progressive management of open surgical repair of Achilles tendon rupture. J Athl Train 1994;29(4):349–51.

29. Suchak AA, Spooner C, Reid DC, et al. Postoperative rehabilitation protocols for Achilles tendon ruptures: a meta-analysis. Clin Orthop Rel Res 2006;445:216–21.

30. Watson TW, Jurist KA, Yang KH, et al. The strength of Achilles tendon repair: an in vitro study of the biomechanical behavior in human cadaver tendons. Foot Ankle Int 1995;16(4):191–5.

31. Jaakkola JI, Hutton WC, Beskin JL, et al. Achilles tendon rupture repair: biomechanical comparison of the triple bundle technique versus the Krakow locking loop technique. Foot Ankle Int 2000;21(1):14–17.

32. Jaakkola JI, Beskin JL, Griffith LH, et al. Early ankle motion after triple bundle technique repair vs. casting for acute Achilles tendon rupture. Foot Ankle Int 2001;22(12):979–84.

33. Krackow KA, Thomas SC, Jones LC. A new stitch for ligament-tendon fixation. Brief note. J Bone Joint Surg [Am] 1986;68(5):764–6.

34. Maffulli N, Tallon C, Wong J, et al. Early weightbearing and ankle mobilization after open repair of acute midsubstance tears of the Achilles tendon. Am J Sports Med 2003;31(5):692–700.

35. Wills CA, Washburn S, Caiozzo V, et al. Achilles tendon rupture. A review of the literature comparing surgical versus nonsurgical treatment. Clin Orthop Rel Res 1986;(207):156–63.

36. Stanec S, Stanec Z, Delimar D, et al. A composite forearm free flap for the secondary repair of the ruptured Achilles tendon. Plast Reconstr Surg 1999;104(5):1409–12.

37. Calliada F, Orlandi S, Pellegrini F. [Clinico-statistical review of 74 cases of sub-cutaneous rupture of the Achilles tendon]. Chir Ital 1979;31(5):1018–25.

9

Rehabilitation After Acute Ruptures of the Achilles Tendon

Anish R. Kadakia, Kelly Short PT, and Mark S. Myerson

Postoperative regimens after Achilles tendon rupture can be broadly categorized as delayed rehabilitation or early functional rehabilitation. Delayed rehabilitation utilizes cast treatment to immobilize the tendon. This common postoperative practice after open Achilles repair includes a 4- to 6-week period in a non–weight bearing, short leg cast that begins in equinus and is gradually brought to neutral. Full weight bearing is typically permitted at 4 to 6 weeks in a short leg cast, after which the cast is removed and physio therapy is begun.[1–6]

Prolonged immobilization, although fully protecting the repair from traumatic rerupture and gapping at the repair site, is associated with multiple complications such as arthrofibrosis, muscle atrophy, deep vein thrombosis, adhesions, and articular cartilage degeneration.[7–9] Immobilization is causally related to a decrease in muscle size, a decrease in the force-generating capacity per unit area, and interstitial fibrosis.[7,10] Immobilization impacts the tendon itself, resulting in lower tensile strength and strain at failure with altered physiologic characteristics.[11,12]

The goal of postoperative care is to protect the repair while providing the optimum conditions for regeneration. A strong body of evidence suggests that postoperative casting and immobilization does not provide ideal conditions for tendon healing. Gelberman et al.,[13] in a canine model, has shown that early protected passive mobilization after flexor tendon repairs produced tendons with higher ultimate load to failure after 12 weeks compared to those that were immobilized. Enwemeka et al.[14] has demonstrated in a rat model that early functional activity provided increased tendon strength without an increased rerupture rate. Controlled tension on the tendon during the healing phase leads to improved collagen synthesis and fiber orientation, resulting in improved tensile strength.[13,15,16] Clinical studies have demonstrated the detriments of immobilization, documenting a 10% to 20% decrease in the strength of the operative side as compared to normal.[4,17–19]

Many clinical studies emphasize early mobilization as a core component of the postoperative protocol.[8,19–28] Concerns about early postoperative mobilization relate to increased gap formation at the repair site, with associated lengthening and rerupture. Overlengthening leads to functional weakening

J.A. Nunley (ed.), *The Achilles Tendon: Treatment and Rehabilitation*,
DOI: 10.1007/978-1-387-79206-4_9, © Springer Science+Business Media, LLC 2009

secondary to increased excursion distance required to generate tension on the tendon.

Open Surgical Repair

Mortensen and Jensen[19] performed a prospective randomized study evaluating the use of early motion after open repair of an Achilles tendon rupture, compared to their standard 8 weeks of cast immobilization. The postoperative protocol for early motion involved 2 weeks of an equinus splint to allow for wound healing. Patients were then placed in a brace that allowed dorsiflexion to a neutral position for an additional 2 weeks. At 4 weeks postoperatively, weight bearing was allowed with the boot in neutral, and active unloaded range of motion was performed. Normal walking began at 6 weeks. Patients treated with early mobilization had a smaller initial loss in the range of motion, earlier return to work and sports activities, and fewer visible adhesions, and were subjectively more satisfied than the immobilized group. Notably, there was no significant difference with respect to the number of reruptures, tendon elongation (as document by radiographic markers placed intraoperatively), or plantar flexion strength.

Troop et al.[29] evaluated 13 patients with an early motion postoperative regimen following open repair of an acute Achilles tendon rupture. Early passive motion began at an average of 10 days and was monitored by a physical therapist. Active range of motion began at an average of 23 days with weight bearing in a boot at neutral at a mean of 3.5 weeks. The boot was discontinued at an average of 7 weeks. The authors noted only one case of a partial rerupture in a patient who was not compliant with the protocol and returned to jumping activities 10 weeks after surgery. Cybex strength testing noted 92% plantarflexion strength and 88% plantarflexion endurance compared to the normative leg.

Speck and Klaue[8] examined 20 patients after open repair with an aggressive rehabilitation involving weight bearing in a boot at neutral and passive range-of-motion exercises beginning on postoperative day 1. The walking boot was discontinued at 6 weeks with initiation of strengthening exercises. No reruptures, skin necroses, or scar adhesions occurred with this protocol. Evaluation at 12 months postoperative with Cybex dynamometer testing showed no significant differences in the strength or power between the operative and unaffected lower extremities.

Mandelbaum et al.[24] studied 29 patients who underwent open Achilles repair after acute rupture followed by early functional rehabilitation. Postoperatively at 48 to 72 hours, the patients' intraoperative dressings were converted to removable posterior splints that allowed the institution of early range-of-motion exercises. Patients were encouraged to perform 10 to 20 degrees of dorsiflexion and plantarflexion four to five times a day. At 2 weeks, patients were placed into a hinged walking brace that allowed full plantarflexion while blocking dorsiflexion at 10 degrees of equinus. Partial weight bearing was initiated at 2 weeks, with progression to full weight bearing at 4 weeks with the boot in neutral or with a cowboy boot. All patients returned to full sports activity by 12 months. Cybex dynamometer testing showed a mean functional deficit of only 2.9% in strength and 2.3% in power compared to the uninjured leg. No reruptures or skin necroses occurred in these patients. The following case study exemplifies the postoperative protocol.

Case Study 1

A 50-year-old graphic designer without preexisting complaints of pain in the Achilles tendon felt a "pop" in her right lower extremity while playing volleyball. Although the patient was very active in running and biking, she did not typically play volleyball. She was otherwise healthy without complicating systemic or medication factors. A physical exam revealed ecchymosis over the posterior medial Achilles. A palpable defect was noted approximately 4 cm proximal to the Achilles insertion. A Thompson's test was positive with no plantarflexion with gastrocnemius squeeze. The patient underwent surgical intervention with an open technique 72 hours after the injury. An open tendon repair was performed with a No. 2 nonabsorbable polyfilament utilizing a stitch technique developed by Krackow et al.[30] in order to create stable internal fixation.[24]

Postoperatively, the patient's leg was placed in a boot, and active unloaded range of motion was initiated four to five times a day. Full weight bearing began at 4 weeks with a dorsiflexion block to neutral. Physical therapy began at 2 weeks and followed the protocol outlined in Table 9.1. Use of the boot was discontinued at 6 weeks, with continued physical therapy. The patient was allowed to return to running at 3 months and did not experience any complications.

Functional Rehabilitation Protocol

Weeks 0 to 2

Following repair of the tendon intraoperatively, the patient is placed into a bulky splint in 20 degrees of plantarflexion in order to minimize swelling and maximize skin perfusion.[31] The patient is non–weight bearing on the operative side and is instructed to keep the leg elevated in order to minimize wound complications.

Week 2

At 2 weeks, the postoperative splint is removed and the patient is placed into a removable cam walker. The goal at this time is to allow the patient to begin weight bearing with the ankle held in 20 degrees of plantarflexion. This can be accomplished by placing a (–)20 degrees of dorsiflexion block in the boot itself or by placing wedges in the boot to place the ankle in 20 degrees of plantarflexion with the boot itself at neutral. Placing the boot itself in 20 degrees equinus leads to a significant disturbance in the patient's gait. The patient is effectively ambulating with an equinus contracture and lengthened lower extremity. This can lead to knee pain secondary to the recurvatum thrust placed on the knee. Also, contralateral hip and low back pain can ensue secondary to the significant leg-length discrepancy. To prevent this, the boot should be fit in a neutral dorsiflexion block, allowing full plantarflexion and utilizing heel lifts to place the ankle in 20 degrees of plantarflexion to protect the repair.

Table 9.1. Postoperative functional rehabilitation protocol after acute Achilles tendon rupture.

Week	Weight-bearing status	Range-of-motion (ROM) exercise	Strength exercise	Therapy adjuncts	Aqua therapy
0–2	Non–weight bearing	Splinted	None	None	None
2	Progressive, partial in boot with wedges to maintain 20 degrees of equinus	Dorsiflexion (−20 degrees)/plantar-flexion (full); circumduction (both directions); two sets of 20 repetitions each exercise	Isometric inversion/eversion; toe curls with towel and weight; hamstring curls in prone with boot; two sets of 10 repetitions for each exercise	Cryotherapy; soft tissue/scar mobilization	None
3	Progress to weight bearing as tolerated	Continue ROM from week 2; begin ankle stretch to neutral with towel	Isometric inversion/eversion and dorsiflexion/plantarflexion, two sets of 20 repetitions; light band-resisted exercises begin, two sets of 10 repetitions; prone knee flexion, two sets of 10 repetitions; stationary bike with boot at low resistance	Cryotherapy; soft tissue/scar mobilization	No weight bearing utilizing a flotation device; range of motion, walking, and running initiated
4–6	Full in brace with wedges to maintain 10 degrees of equinus	Continue ROM from previous weeks; ankle stretch with towel with knee extended and at 40 degrees of flexion	Continue isometric exercise as outlined in week 3; increase resistive band exercise at three sets of 20 repetitions; hamstring curls with light resistance at three sets of 20 repetitions	Cross-fiber massage begun; ultrasound, iontophoresis, and electrical stimulation to decrease inflammation and scar formation	Continue therapy as outlined in week 3
6–8	Progress to shoe weight bearing as tolerated with a 5- degree wedge	Continued stretching as previously outlined	Stationary bike without boot with increased resistance; continued isotonic and isometric exercises; weight shifting and unilateral balance exercise seated on therapeutic ball; closed chain Partial Weight Bearing (PWB) strengthening of plantar flexors (0 degrees to full plantarflexion); seated heel raises, and hamstring curl with light resistance; open chain strengthening with medium resistive band; begin stair stepper with involved limb only	Soft tissue mobilization; modalities to control edema and pain	Excellent for initiation of weight bearing in obese patients; walking in water and standing heel raises (waist deep or greater); flutter kick with kickboard

| 8–10 | Weight bearing in shoe full time with heel 5-degree wedge | Continue as needed to ensure neutral dorsiflexion is achieved | Stationary bike with increasing resistance; eccentric focused strengthening of plantar flexors; band-resisted exercises advancing to heavy band as tolerated; progress to standing heel raises; progress to standing balance exercise in tandem and single limb support (close eyes to increase difficulty) | Continued as needed | Continue as outlined above; initiate plyometrics and conditioning exercises |

A formal physical therapy program is then begun under the direct supervision of the therapist. Range-of-motion exercises from 20 degrees plantarflexion to full plantarflexion are started, along with circumduction (both clockwise and counterclockwise). Strengthening exercises with isometric inversion and eversion, with the ankle held in 20 degrees plantarflexion, are begun. Toe curls with towels and weight along with hamstring curls are initiated (Fig. 9.1). All exercises are performed in two sets with 10 repetitions per set. Cryotherapy is utilized in order to minimize swelling.

Week 3

Weight bearing in the boot with heel lifts places the ankle in 10 degrees of plantarflexion. Soft tissue and scar mobilization is performed. Initiation of a stationary bike with the boot in place at low resistance comes next. Aqua therapy may be implemented using a flotation device to prevent weight bearing on the operative leg. Range-of-motion exercises are continued from week 2 in order to increase dorsiflexion to neutral using a strap or towel (Fig. 9.2).

Strength exercises are continued with the addition of isometric dorsiflexion and plantarflexion exercises. Light resisted band inversion, eversion, dorsiflexion, and plantarflexion exercises are implemented over the course of week 3 (Fig. 9.3). The frequency is increased to two sets with 20 repetitions per set.

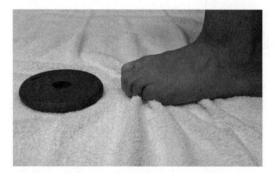

Fig. 9.1. Toe curls utilizing a towel and weight

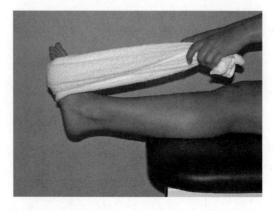

Fig. 9.2. A towel is used to gently perform a dorsiflexion stretch to the Achilles tendon

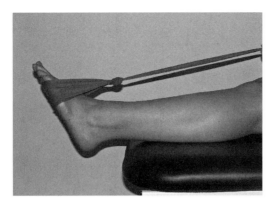

Fig. 9.3. Resistive band exercise for plantarflexion strength

Week 4

Weight bearing in the boot at the neutral position is initiated. Gentle, cross-fiber massage to the Achilles is performed along with ultrasound, phonophoresis, and electrical stimulation to decrease inflammation and adhesion formation. The stationary bike and aqua therapy continue as outlined in week 3.

Continued stretching of the Achilles tendon is performed using a towel. Stretching while standing is initiated only if the patient has not achieved neutral dorsiflexion. Strengthening continues, and the resistance of the bands is increased. Hamstring curls are continued to facilitate gastrocnemius muscle strength without flexing the ankle and stressing the repair. Exercise now increases to three sets with 20 repetitions per set.

Week 6

The use of the boot is now discontinued, and weight bearing is permitted in a shoe with a 5-degree heel lift. Modalities and soft tissue mobilization are continued as outlined in week 4.

A significant increase in patient activity is now initiated. Use of a stationary bicycle is allowed without the boot, and resistance is increased as tolerated along with use of a stair stepper. Closed chain strengthening of the gastroc-soleus complex is initiated using seated heel raises, and hamstring curls with light resistance. Gait training with a concentration on weight shifting from heel-to-toe and side-to-side shifting begins.

Aqua therapy is progressed. This is ideal for obese patients, as it decreases the tensile stress on the repair. Aqua therapy also helps athletes maintain their conditioning. Therapy is performed in water that is at least waist deep and begins with standing heel raises and walking. Flutter kicking with a kickboard is begun, while fins are utilized to increase resistance.

Week 8

Therapy is continued with a focus on increasing the strength of the gastroc-soleus complex. Isotonic exercises are continued with an increasing eccentric bias. Standing balance exercises in tandem is begun and progresses to single leg support (Fig. 9.4). Aqua therapy is continued with the addition of plyometrics in waist-deep water. Plyometrics involves the lengthening of a muscle, followed by its immediate contraction. This results in a very powerful force that can injure the muscle and should be performed under the supervision of a therapist.

Week 10

The heel lift is now no longer required (Table 9.2.). Squats are begun with moderated resistance in order to prevent excessive dorsiflexion of the ankle. Standing heel raises are continued with a focus on single limb concentric and eccentric strengthening. Resisted walking is initiated using free motion machines, pulleys, and bands. Use of an elliptical trainer is excellent for improving strength and range of motion at this time.

Aqua therapy is progressed to include aerobic conditioning. In athletes, this type of therapy focuses on plyometrics. Plyometric exercise, which is excellent to increase the explosive power of the athlete, is unsafe to perform outside of the pool.

Week 12

Therapy is focused on graduating the patient to normal activity. The initiation of jogging and plyometric training outside of the pool is begun if the patient is able to perform a single limb heel rise 10 times with a low pain rating. Aqua therapy is continued as needed in obese patients who may have a slightly delayed recovery.

Achillon® Surgical Repair

Open surgical repair, although reliable in obtaining excellent functional results, carries the risk of wound complications that is avoided by nonoperative management. To maximize the benefits of open surgical repair in conjunction

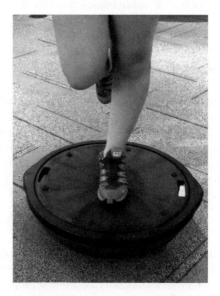

Fig. 9.4. Use of a balance board to perform a single limb support focusing on both strength and proprioceptive training

Table 9.2. Functional rehabilitation protocol following surgical repair of an acute Achilles tendon rupture

Week	Weight-bearing status	Range-of-motion (ROM) exercise	Strength exercise	Therapy adjuncts	Aqua therapy
10–12	Weight bearing in shoe without lift	Standing stretch past neutral dorsiflexion	Continue stationary bike; squats with moderated resistance; standing balance exercise—use perturbation (band resist, ball toss); standing heel raises (eccentric and concentric strengthening); resisted walking (free motion machine, bands, and pulleys); elliptical trainer	Continue as needed	Continue as outlined above
12–14	Weight bearing in shoe without lift	Full range of motion	Continue stationary bike; balance exercise unless symmetrical bilaterally; unilateral heel raises (eccentric strengthening); if able to perform 10 single limb heel rise AND low pain rating may progress to stair stepper, plyometrics, and jogging	Continue as needed	Continue as outlined above if needed

with minimizing the wound complication rate, percutaneous and limited open procedures have been developed.[9,32-34]

A primary concern following percutaneous repair is the strength of the fixation and its effect on postoperative rehabilitation and outcome. Buchgraber and Passler[21] performed a retrospective review of 48 patients who had undergone percutaneous repair utilizing a 1.2-mm PDS cord. Postoperatively, patients were treated with casting (18 patients) for 6 weeks or functional rehabilitation (30 patients). Functional rehabilitation consisted of an anterior splint in 10 to 20 degrees of plantarflexion for a mean of 2.7 days, which was then converted to a special shoe (Adimed-Stabil Ortotech, Gauting, Germany) with a 3-cm heel lift. Patients were allowed to weight bear immediately after obtaining the shoe, and isometric muscle exercises began. An isokinetic regimen started at 4 weeks. Patients in the functional group had a reduced return-to-work time and a superior visual analogue scale outcome score. No significant overlengthening of the tendon occurred in the functional group, as evidenced by no significant increase in the amount of dorsiflexion in the functional group compared to the casted group. One case of rerupture was noted in the functional group in a patient who disregarded postoperative protocol and played tennis too soon. Cybex II testing did not reveal any significant differences between the two groups with respect to plantarflexion strength. The authors do not recommend the use of cast treatment following percutaneous repair, given the superior subjective outcome and decreased convalescence period associated with functional rehab.

The use of the Achillon® system (Newdeal SA, Lyon, France) allows the benefit of minimally invasive repair without the risk of permanent injury to the sural nerve.[21,22,25,27,35–38] The system initially described by Assal et al.[22] uses unique instrumentation that places the suture underneath the paratenon, thus minimizing risk to the sural nerve. A small longitudinal or transverse incision is made directly over the rupture to visualize the rupture and ensure tendon apposition during tying of the three sutures used for fixation. Following this repair, patients were treated with a program of functional rehabilitation. Postoperatively, patients' legs were placed in a boot locked in 30 degrees of plantarflexion with partial weight bearing for 2 weeks. Stationary biking and unloaded active range-of-motion exercises started at 3 weeks with full weight bearing in the boot at the neutral position. Use of the orthosis was discontinued at 8 weeks. Eighty-two patients were followed for a mean of 26 months. No patients suffered a thrombosis, embolus, superficial or deep infection, or sural neuritis. Three patients suffered rerupture (3.7%), two of which were secondary to falls because the patients were noncompliant and removed the orthosis early at 2 and 3 weeks, respectively. All patients returned to their previous work and sports activities at the same level of participation, including five members of the Swiss national teams for fencing, martial arts, and soccer. No significant difference in the mean number of single limb hops was demonstrated. No significant difference in the mean concentric peak torque was demonstrated between the operative and normal side.

Calder and Saxby[25] evaluated the use of the Achillon system with postoperative functional rehabilitation in 46 patients. All patients were followed a minimum of 12 months with no reruptures, one superficial wound infection, and two patients with transient sural neuritis. Postoperatively, patients were placed in an orthosis locked in 20 degrees of plantarflexion for 2 weeks. Beginning at 3 weeks, free range of motion to neutral and an active physiotherapy program were begun. The orthosis was discontinued at 6 weeks, and jogging was restricted for 3 months. All patients had full dorsiflexion of the ankle and returned to full sports activities at 6 months.

The use of minimally invasive techniques does not preclude the use of functional rehabilitation following operative repair. The advantage of minimally invasive techniques is that the small incision utilized allows an earlier start of range-of-motion exercises without a significant risk of wound complications or delayed healing. The following case study exemplifies the rehabilitation following use of the Achillon system.

Case Study 2

A 21-year-old collegiate football player felt an acute "pop" in his right lower extremity during practice. Physical examination was consistent with an acute midsubstance Achilles tendon rupture. To decrease the risk of wound complications in a high-level athlete and to decrease the risk of reruptures, operative intervention was performed with the Achillon system. A 1-cm transverse incision at the level of the rupture was utilized along with No. 1 nonabsorbable polyfilament for fixation. Postoperatively, the patient was placed in a splint in 20 degrees of plantarflexion in order to maximize skin perfusion over the Achilles.[31] The patient underwent functional rehabilitation as outlined for patients who have undergone open repair; however, the splint was discontinued at 1 week, and earlier range-of-motion therapy begun, because of a minimal risk of wound complications. At 6 months, the patient could perform the same number of single heel rises with his injured leg as compared to his uninjured leg, and he returned to full sports activity. The patient was completely satisfied and felt that no decrease in the level of competitive play occurred.

Insertional Achilles Rupture

A less common condition is that associated with an Achilles "sleeve" avulsion, or insertional rupture of the Achilles tendon. This type of rupture is almost always associated with chronic inflammation and degeneration at the Achilles insertion.[26] This type of rupture does not have sufficient distal soft tissue to facilitate a direct tendon-to-tendon repair. The degeneration and poor quality of the distal stump of the Achilles along with the less secure fixation of the tendon to the calcaneus either with transosseous suture or suture anchors require a modification of the functional rehabilitation protocol in order to prevent reruptures, as in the following case study.

Case Study 3

A 27-year-old professional baseball player with preexisting insertional Achilles tendonitis suffered an acute injury to the affected lower extremity. Examination was consistent with an Achilles tendon sleeve rupture. Magnetic resonance imaging was consistent with an insertional rupture of the Achilles with insufficient distal soft tissue for primary tendon-to-tendon repair. Minimally invasive techniques are not appropriate for this type of rupture, and formal open repair using a J-type incision is very useful. Operative repair was performed with resection of the prominent superior calcaneal tuberosity and fixation of the tendon to the broad cancellous surface with a suture anchor. The diseased portion of the tendon was resected, and the remaining distal stump was repaired as an augmentation once the tendon was secured to the calcaneus.

Rehabilitation following this injury requires protection of the repair, given the poor quality of the tendon and less rigid fixation compared to a standard midsubstance tear. Postoperatively, the splint is removed at 2 weeks and the use of a cast or orthosis with the ankle in fixed 20 degrees of plantarflexion with partial weight bearing is used for 2 weeks. At week 4, the ankle is allowed range of motion using a hinged orthosis with a neutral dorsiflexion block using wedges to place the ankle in 10 degrees of plantarflexion; weight bearing as tolerated is permitted. Therapy starts for active unloaded range of motion, cryotherapy, and soft tissue and scar mobilization. At 6 weeks, the therapeutic protocol for a standard Achilles rupture is now initiated, effectively delaying the rehabilitation by 4 weeks. The boot is discontinued at 10 weeks. Given that this patient was a high-level athlete, aqua therapy was aggressively utilized to maximize functional recovery without increasing the risk of rerupture.

Conclusion

Functional rehabilitation offers the advantages associated with early range of motion following tendon repair, with increased strength of the healed tendon, minimal skin necrosis, and lack of arthrofibrosis.[8,19,24,29] There has not been an associated increase in rerupture with early range-of-motion protocols compared to immobilized patients.[8,19,24,29] Following functional rehabilitation, patients have been able to perform nearly symmetric strength and power testing, in contrast to a 10% to 20% deficit with cast immoblization.[4,8,17–19,24] The overall superiority with respect to outcome without a significant rerupture rate supports the use of functional rehabilitation over cast immobilization after open repair.

References

1. Crolla R, van Leeuwen D, van Ramshort B, van der Wenken C. Acute rupture of the tendo calcaneus. Surgical repair with functional after treatment. Acta Orthop Belg 1987;53:492–4.
2. Inglis A, Scott W, Sculco T. Ruptures of the tendo Achilles. J Bone Joint Surg 1970;58:990–3.
3. Kellam J, Hunter G, McElwain J. Review of the operative treatment of Achilles tendon rupture. Clin Orthop Rel Res 1985;201:80–3.
4. Haji A, Sahai A, Symes A, Vyas J. Percutaneous versus open tendo achillis repair. Foot Ankle Int 2004;25(4):215–8.
5. Goren D, Ayalon M, Nyska M. Isokinetic strength and endurance after percutaneous and open surgical repair of Achilles tendon ruptures. Foot Ankle Int 2005;26(4):286–90.
6. Wills C, Washburn S, Caiozzo V, Prietto C. Achilles tendon rupture. A review of the literature comparing surgical versus nonsurgical treatment. Clin Orthop Rel Res 1986;207:156–63.
7. Booth F. Physiologic and biochemical effects of immobilization muscle. Clin Orthop Rel Res 1987;219:15–20.
8. Speck M, Klaue K. Early full weightbearing and functional treatment after surgical repair of acute Achilles tendon rupture. Am J Sports Med 1998;26(6):789–93.
9. Ma G, Griffith T. Percutaneous repair of acute closed ruptured Achilles tendon. Clin Orthop Rel Res 1977;128:247–55.
10. Qin L, Appell H, Chan K, Mafulli N. Electrical stimulation prevents immobilization atrophy in skeletal muscle of rabbits. Arch Phys Med Rehabil 1997;78(5):512–7.
11. Akeson W, Woo S, Amiel D, Coutts R, Daniel D. The connective tissue response to immobility: biochemical changes in periarticular connective tissue of the immobilized rabbit knee. Clin Orthop Rel Res 1973;93:356–62.
12. Yamamoto E, Hayashi K, Yamamoto N. Mechanical properties of collagen fascicles from stress-shielded patellar tendons in the rabbit. Clin Biomech 1999;14:418–25.
13. Gelberman R, Woo S, Lothringer K, Akeson W, Amiel D. Effects of early intermittent passive mobilization on healing canine flexor tendons. J Hand Surg [Am] 1982;7(2):170–5.
14. Enwemeka C, Spielholz N, Nelson A. The effect of early functional activities on experimentally tenotomized Achilles tendons in rats. Am J Phys Med Rehabil 1988;68:264–9.
15. Gelberman R, Menon J, Gonsalves M, Akeson W. The effects of mobilization on the vascularization of healing flexor tendons in dogs. Clin Orthop Rel Res 1980;153:283–9.
16. Kellet J. Acute soft tissue injuries—a review of the literature. Med Sci Sports Exerc 1986;18:489–500.
17. Bradley J, Tibone J. Percutaneous and open surgical repairs of Achilles tendon ruptures. A comparative study. Am J Sports Med 1990;118:188–95.
18. Nistor L. Surgical and non-surgical treatment of Achilles tendon rupture. J Bone Joint Surg 1981;63:394–9.

19. Mortensen N, Jensen P. Early motion of the ankle after operative treatment of a rupture of the Achilles tendon. A prospective, randomized clinical and radiographic study. J Bone Joint Surg 1999;81(7):983–90.
20. McComis GP, Nawoczenzki DA, Dehaven KE. Functional bracing for rupture of the Achilles tendon. Clinical results and analysis of ground-reaction forces and temporal data. J Bone Joint Surg 1997;79(12):1799–808.
21. Buchgraber A, Passler HH. Percutaneous repair of Achilles tendon rupture: immobilization versus functional postoperative treatment. Clin Orthop Rel Res 1997;341:113–22.
22. Assal M, Jung M, Stern R, Rippinstein P, Delmi M, Hoffmeyer P. Limited open repair of Achilles tendon ruptures: a technique with a new instrument and findings of a prospective multicenter study. J Bone Joint Surg 2002;84(2):161–70.
23. Shilders E, Bismil Q, Metcalf R, Marynissen H. Clinical tip: Achilles tendon repair with accelerated rehabilitation program. Foot Ankle Int 2005;26(5):412–5.
24. Mandelbaum BR, Myerson MS, Robert F. Achilles tendon ruptures. A new method of repair, early range of motion, and functional rehabilitation. Am J Sports Med 1995;23(4):392–5.
25. Calder J, Saxby T. Early, active rehabilitation following mini-open repair of Achilles tendon rupture: a prospective study. Br J Sports Med 2005;39:857–9.
26. Bibbo C, Anderson RB, Davis WH, Agnone M. Repair of the Achilles tendon sleeve avulsion: quantitative and functional evaluation of a transcalcaneal suture technique. Foot Ankle Int 2003;24(7):539–44.
27. Calder J, Saxby T. Independent evaluation of a recently described Achilles tendon repair technique. Foot Ankle Int 2006;27(2):93–6.
28. Gorschewsky O, Pitzl M, Putz A, Klakow A, Neumann W. Percutaneous repair of acute Achilles tendon rupture. Foot Ankle Int 2004;25(4):219–24.
29. Troop RL, Losse GM, Lane JG, Robertson DB, Hastings PS, Howard ME. Early motion after repair of Achilles tendon rupture. Foot Ankle Int 1995;16(11):705–9.
30. Krackow K, Thomas S, Jones L. A new stitch for ligament-tendon fixation. Brief note. J Bone Joint Surg 1986;68:764–6.
31. Poynton A, O'Rourke K. An analysis of skin perfusion over the Achilles tendon in varying degrees of plantarflexion. Foot Ankle Int 2001;22(7):572–4.
32. Delponte P, Potier L, de Poulpiquet P, Buisson P. Treatment of subcutaneous ruptures of the Achilles tendon by percutaneous tenorrhaphy. Rev Chir Orthop 1992;78:404–7.
33. Fitz Gibbons R, Hefferon J, Hill J. Percutaneous Achilles tendon repair. Am J Sports Med 1993;21:724–7.
34. Kakiuchi M. A combined open and percutaneous technique for repair of tendo Achillis. Comparison with open repair. J Bone Joint Surg 1995;77B:60–3.
35. Aracil J, Pina A, Lozano J, Torro V, Escriba I. Percutaneous suture of Achilles tendon ruptures. Foot Ankle 1992;13:350–1.
36. Rowley D, Scotland T. Rupture of the Achilles tendon treated by a simple operative procedure. Injury 1982;14:252–4.
37. Steele G, Harter R, Ting A. Comparison of functional ability following percutaneous and open surgical repairs of acutely ruptured tendons. J Sport Rehabil 1993;2(115–127).
38. FitzGibbons R, Hefferon J, Hill J. Percutaneous Achilles tendon repair. Am J Sports Med 1993;21:724–7.

Section III

Chronic Injuries

10

Treatment of the Chronic Elongated Achilles Tendon with Anatomic Reconstruction

Beat Hintermann and Markus Knupp

Although ruptures of the Achilles tendon are relatively common, a delayed or missed diagnosis by the primary treating physician is a frequent occurrence. Inglis and Sculco[1] reported that 38 (23%) of 167 Achilles tendon ruptureswere initially misdiagnosed. This consequently leads to an inappropriate primary treatment that results in an incomplete or deficient healing, typically associated with elongation and either a partial or complete chronic rupture of the tendon. Similar disabling conditions may also result from a degenerative disease of the tendon.

Treatment of the resulting condition is often demanding, and bridging the resulting gap may require extensive surgical approaches. For this purpose, various procedures have been described that can be divided into three groups:

1. Primary repair, which may be possible for defects up to 2 cm
2. Augmentation with either a fascia advancement (V-Y-plasty or gastroc-soleus fascia turn-down graft) or a local tendon transfer
3. Synthetic or allograft reconstruction

Descriptions of tendon grafts include reconstruction with the peroneus brevis tendon,[2,3] the flexor digitorum longus tendon,[4] or the flexor hallucis longus tendon.[5–8] The disadvantage of these procedures is that other healthy structures (e.g., a flexor tendon) need to be sacrificed. Loss of the harvested structures may consequently lead to residual ankle instability and gait changes with loss of push-off power. Techniques for anatomic reconstruction have been described by Abraham and Pankovich,[9] who suggested a V-Y advancement, and by Bosworth,[10] who proposed a turn-down procedure. Both of these techniques may be complemented with a plantaris tendon enforcement. Finally, some attempts have been made to use allografts of synthetic and biologic materials.[11] There are, however, no long-term studies published on these techniques.

Etiology of Chronic Rupture

In contrast to an acute mechanical failure of the tendon, which usually correlates with an injury, a spontaneous rupture of the Achilles tendon is

J.A. Nunley (ed.), *The Achilles Tendon: Treatment and Rehabilitation*,
DOI: 10.1007/978-1-387-79206-4_10, © Springer Science+Business Media, LLC 2009

more difficult to detect. It can be associated with a multitude of disorders such as inflammatory and autoimmune conditions,[12] genetically determined collagen abnormalities,[13] infectious diseases,[14,15] and neurologic conditions. Any of these underlying diseases may predispose the tendon to spontaneous rupture following minor trauma.[16] An additional contributing factor may be the decreased blood flow in the tendon with increasing age. This is supported by the fact that the area of the Achilles tendon that is typically prone to rupture is relatively avascular compared to the rest of the tendon.[17,18]

Injections of corticosteroids have been found to increase the risk of rupture of the tendon.[18] The antiinflammatory and analgesic properties of corticosteroids may mask the symptoms of tendon damage, inducing individuals to maintain high levels of activity even when the tendon is damaged. Corticosteroids furthermore interfere with healing and intratendinous injection of corticosteroids results in a weakening of the tendon for as many as 14 days.[19]The disruption is directly related to collagen necrosis, and restoration of the strength of the tendon is attributable to the formation of an acellular amorphous mass of collagen. Fluoroquinolone antibiotics, such as ciprofloxacin, have recently been implicated in the etiology of tendon ruptures.[20]

Kannus and Jozsa[21]noted pathologic alterations in all of the 891 spontaneously ruptured tendons. All probes studied showed histologic changes, 97% of which were degenerative. The most common degenerative lesion found was hypoxic degeneration, with alterations in the size and shape of the mitochondria, abnormal tenocyte nuclei, and occasional intracytoplasmic or mitochondrial calcium deposit. In advanced degeneration, hypoxic or lipid vacuoles were observed. Aberrant collagen fibers were also seen, with abnormal variations in the diameter, angulation, splitting, and disintegration of the fibers. The authors also noted vascular changes, mostly luminal narrowing due to hypertrophy of the arterial intima and media, in vessels of the tendon and paratenon in 62% of the 891 ruptures. Alterations in the blood flow and subsequent hypoxia, as well as an impaired metabolism, may have been factors in the development of the degenerative changes observed in the ruptured tendons.

All these factors contribute to a poor tissue quality and reduced healing capacity of the tendon, making any treatment of a chronically ruptured Achilles tendon challenging.

Diagnosis

The most common method of diagnosis for Achilles tendinopathy is a thorough assessment of the patient's history and a careful clinical examination that identifies any pain and tenderness within the tendon. The examination should ascertain whether the patient has pain during physical activity or at rest. The physical examination should be conducted with the patient prone, with the feet hanging off the edge of the examination table (Fig.10.1). The entire substance of the gastrocnemius-soleus myotendinous complex should be palpated while the ankle is gently put through active and passive ranges of motion. Calf atrophy, a common finding with chronic Achilles disease, can be recognized by comparing maximal girth measurements on the involved and noninvolved sides. Tenderness, crepitation, warmth, swelling, nodularity, and substance defects should be noted.

With either a partial or complete chronic rupture, the physical examination reveals findings such as a localized, tender area of swelling that occasionally involves an area of nodularity, or a painless defect (Fig. 10.2) . Chronic rupture of the Achilles tendon often leads to elongation of the soleus or the gastrocnemius complex. Plantarflexion power of the triceps muscle may be diminished, but can be preserved to some extent. In most instances, the patient is able to perform a single heel raise, however, only to a certain extent and over a short period of time (as compared with the unaffected contralateral side). Comparing both the affected and the unaffected contralateral foot, while the patient is sitting with the feet hanging off the edge of the examination table, an increased passive dorsiflexion of the ankle may indicate an elongation of the soleus complex. If this finding persists while the knee is fully extended, the gastrocnemius complex is also elongated (Silfverskiöld test). If so, a hyperextension at the knee can often be seen while the patient is standing on both feet.

The two modalities that give the best images of the Achilles tendon are sonography and magnetic resonance imaging (MRI) (Fig. 10.3). Recent

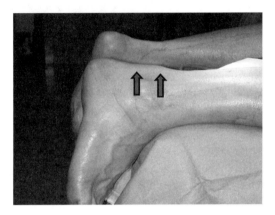

Fig. 10.1. While the patient is in a prone position with the feet hanging off the edge of the examination table, inspection from medially or laterally shows thickening or a gap of the tendon (arrows)

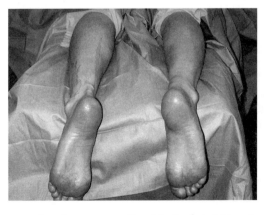

Fig. 10.2. From posterior view, an area of nodularity (asterisk) and a painless defect (arrow) are visible (same patient as in Fig. 10.1)

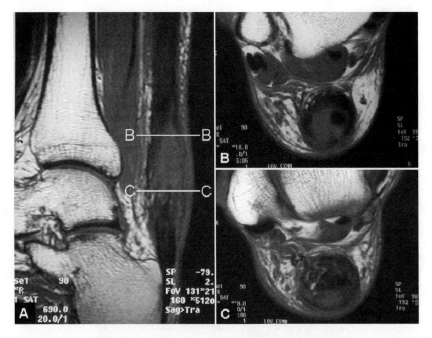

Fig. 10.3. In this 38-year-old soccer player with a trauma 12 months previously, magnetic resonance imaging (MRI) revealed a complete rupture (A) with an extended defect of the deep portion of the Achilles tendon close to its distal insertion (B), whereas the superficial layer was ruptured more proximally (C), which had hidden the rupture by clinical investigation. The lines BB and CC indicate the level of the transversal plane shown in Fig. b and c respectively

refinements in both technologies have tremendously improved our ability to image pathologic changes in tendons. Sonography is the most reliable technique to determine the thickness of the Achilles tendon and the size of the gap after a complete rupture (Fig. 10.4). It has also the potential for dynamic examination. It does, however, require substantial experience to learn how to operate the probe and to interpret the images correctly.

Magnetic resonance imaging is superior in detecting incomplete tendon ruptures and the evaluation of various stages of chronic degenerative changes. It can also be used to monitor tendon healing when a recurrent partial rupture is suspected. Magnetic resonance imaging may not give a complete diagonosis, but it usually helps to identify the causes in which surgery is nessecary.

In most cases radiographs do not add more information and are usually not necessary to make the diagnosis. They may, however, demonstrate calcification within the tendon and can be used to exclude avulsions of the posterior calcaneal tuberosity.

Postsurgical histopathology can be used in selected cases to confirm the diagnosis. This is, however, the only way to be diagnostically certain of the underlying abnormalities.

Indications and Contraindications for Surgical Reconstruction

The local chronically affected tissue has only poor healing capacity, and the affected area usually lies in the watershed area of the tendon.[17]Therefore,

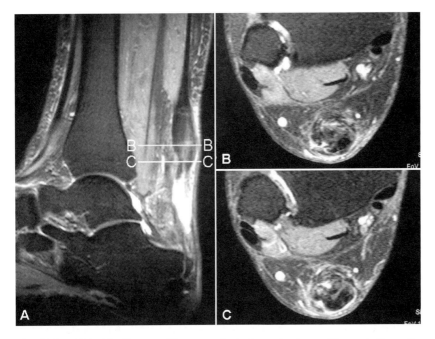

Fig. 10.4. (A) In this 43–year-old runner who had sustained an ankle sprain 9 months prior, MRI revealed an incomplete rupture of the Achilles tendon. (B,C) The gap was filled with hypertrophic scar tissue, which led to the clinical diagnosis of tendonitis

surgical reconstruction of chronic midsubstance Achilles tendon ruptures should be considered in all cases, as nonoperative treatment is unlikely to lead to a satisfying functional outcome. In patients with contraindications for operative treatment, conservative treatment may be considered. The pain may be lessened with high-top shoes, boots, or braces. In most cases, however, conservative treatment will not restore the loss of push-off strength resulting from the elongated tendon.

Preoperative Considerations

Some patients may report a history of cortisone injections to treat the symptoms. This history needs to be taken into consideration when planning the reconstruction as it may have contributed to tendon degeneration. Other problematic conditions include systemic diseases (diabetes mellitus, seronegative inflammatory disease, spondyloarthropathies, or sarcoidosis) and previous infections in the area. The surgeon needs to assess all risk factors very carefully so as not to put the result of his intervention at risk. This is also the case for patients with tobacco use or chronic arterial or venous disease. Patients with severe vascular disease and with sensorimotor deficits, such as peripheral neuropathy or Parkinson's disease, should be excluded from surgical treatment.

Surgical Techniques

With the patient in the prone position, both legs are prepped and draped in the sterile field to determine the appropriate resting tension and in case the plantaris tendon of the contralateral foot is required.[22]

A posteromedial incision is made (Fig. 10.5) , and the sural nerve identified and retracted. Usually most of the paratenon needs to be excised as it may be thickened or scarred. The tendon is then meticulously debrided, removing all macroscopically diseased tissue, and subsequently the length of the resulting gap is measured. Finally, the procedure is determined (e.g., end-to-end suture, V-Y lengthening, or turndown procedure in combination with a plantaris tendon transfer). Defects of less than 2 cm can usually be addressed with an end-to-end repair, especially if the patient is treated within 3 months of the injury. For gaps exceeding 2 cm, a gap-spanning procedure is usually necessary not to risk an early rerupture or an equinus foot position.

Postoperative Management

A compressive dressing and a splint are maintained for 2 to 5 days to diminish swelling. The tendon reconstruction is then protected in a short leg, partial weight-bearing cast in 10 degrees of equinus. After 2 weeks the cast is changed in order to allow suture removal. The duration of the immobilization in the cast is determined by the amount of gastrocnemius atrophy and the amount of time that the tendon has been ruptured. Usually tendons that have been ruptured for over more than 6 months require a longer period of time in the cast. If a good primary strength of the reconstructed tendon is achieved, the cast is removed after 6 weeks and full weight bearing in a commercially available supportive shoe with an augmented heel (Künzli®, Windisch, Switzerland) is permitted. Additionally the patient is referred to a rehabilitation program for strengthening and gait training 8 weeks postoperatively. However, athletic activities are restricted for at least 6 months after surgery, as in the following case study.

Case Study

A 52-year-old patient sustained a rupture of his left Achilles tendon while practicing volleyball. A percutaneous suture was done, and the foot was then

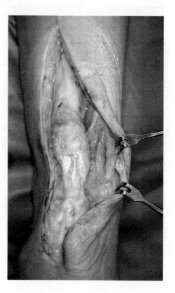

Fig. 10.5. A longitudinal incision on the medial aspect of the tendon is used to expose the scarred tendon and the defect. This enables removing the whole scar until regular tendon tissue is present on both the distal and proximal stump

immobilized in a cast in 20 degrees of plantarflexion for 2 weeks, and then in 10 degrees of plantarflexion for the next 2 weeks, and thereafter in neutral position for 4 additional weeks.

Despite intensive rehabilitation training, loss of triceps power persisted, and the patient complained of pain while walking. Running and other demanding sports activities were not possible.

After 14 months, clinical investigation revealed atrophy of his left calf, rising-up of the left heel was not possible, and there was a significant loss of power compared with the contralateral foot. Palpation of the Achilles tendon revealed a gap of about 3 cm above the tuber calcanei. Magnetic resonance imaging showed a defect of more than 5 cm within the tendon.

Surgical exploration showed a scarred tendon with some sutures left from the previous surgery. The whole scar was excised and the proximal tendon stump was debrided; the distal stump of the tendon was excised because of the poor quality of the tissue. The overall defect was 7 cm long (Fig. 10.6A)

The proximal tendon–muscle complex was further exposed, and a V-shaped incision of the tendon close to the muscular bellies of the gastrocnemius was planned. After sharp dissection of the tendon, it was carefully pulled distalward, with care to preserve its connection to the deep soleus muscle. Thereby an overall lengthening of the tendon–muscle complex of 6 cm was achieved. Side-to-side sutures were done to stabilize the lengthened tendon, resulting in a Y-shaped reconstruction. Then the plantaris tendon that was harvested from the contralateral foot was brought through a horizontal hole of the tuber calcanei. This 4.5-mm hole was previously drilled as close as possible to the posterior aspect of the tuber to get maximal leverage to the axis of rotation.

In addition, a suture anchor (Panalock®, Mitek/Johnson & Johnson) was placed in the center of the posterior aspect of the tuber calcanei. The tendon was pulled distally and then reattached to the tuber calcanei using the suture anchor and some additional transosseus sutures. Then the plantaris tendon was woven through the reconstructed tendon to improve its reattachment to the tuber calcanei and the strength of the reconstructed tendon (Fig. 10.6B).

The postoperative treatment consisted of cast immobilization in 15 degrees of plantar flexion for 2 weeks, followed by neutral foot position for an additional 6 weeks. Rehabilitation training was started after 8 weeks to strengthen the triceps surae and to improve gait and coordination. At 6 months, MRI was done to assess the healing of the reconstructed tendon. It showed a still thickened tendon with an overall continuity between its distal insertion and its proximal V-Y lengthening. At this time, progressive return to all sports activities except contact sports was permitted.

At 1-year follow-up, the patient still experienced a deficit of strength (–36% compared to the contralateral side) as measured by an independent neurologist. However, the patient was very satisfied and considered the regained function to be sufficient for his daily life and sports activities. At 2 years, the deficit of strength was decreased to 18%. The patient finished his first marathon 19 months after surgery and his first triathlon 23 months after surgery.

Preliminary Results

The authors have treated a total of 33 patients with the described procedures. The last follow-up of the patients was after an average of 47 months and so

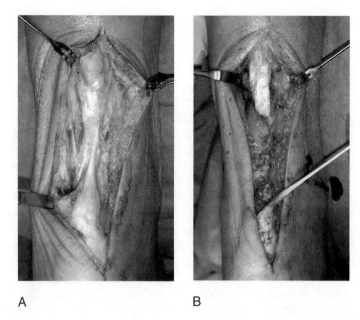

A   B

Fig. 10.6. (A) If the tendon defect is too long for reconstruction by a V-Y lengthening, which is usually the case for defects of more than 7 cm, a turn-down of a 1- to 1.5-cm-wide strip is used to bridge the defect. (B) In this 64-year-old patient, the intact plantaris tendon was dissected at its proximal end and then used for reinforcement of the reconstructed tendon). (From Knupp and Hintermann,[23] with permission of Wolters Kluwer Health.)

far no reruptures have been observed. The clinical evaluation revealed no significant difference in the comparison of the plantarflexion strength of the reconstructed tendon and the uninvolved extremity.[22]

To date the complications were limited to wound healing problems (four cases), which necessitated irrigation and debridement in one case. However, in reconstruction of chronic ruptures of the Achilles tendon there is a considerable risk for wound dehiscence, infection, rerupture, and sural nerve injury. Additionally diminished push-off strength caused by overlengthening of the tendon or a residual equinus position may result secondary to overtightening of the tendon. Another potential complication is a detachment of the tendinous portion of the gastrocnemius-soleus complex from the underlying muscular component with excessive traction during the V-V plasty. We therefore limit the indication for this procedure to defects of less than 6 cm.

The Authors' Experience

Reconstruction of a chronic Achilles tendon rupture may be challenging, as extensile surgical approaches and augmentation are needed in many cases. Often the extent of the defect is only visible intraoperatively, making preoperative planning very difficult. Additionally, previous surgery and cortisone injections often leave behind severely altered soft tissue conditions with only poor healing capacity.

To avoid sacrificing a flexor tendon (i.e., flexor hallucis longus, peroneus brevis) we routinely used a V-Y plasty or a turn-down procedure for reconstruction.

Despite the extensile exposure necessary for the described procedures, we so far have had success with these techniques with only minor complications. However, in cases of severe atrophy or bad soft tissue conditions, particularly in ruptures older than 6 months, surgical treatment may be difficult, and rerupture rates may be high with any of the procedures described. If reconstruction is performed in these cases, it may lead to residual equinus position of the foot. Here it may be advisable to adjust the postoperative treatment with prolongation of the immobilization in a cast. However, we found that even ruptures of 12 months and older achieved a good functional result following surgery with the relevant procedures after an extensile rehabilitation program.

References

1. Inglis AE, Sculco TP. Surgical repair of ruptures of the tendo Achillis. Clin Orthop 1981;156:160–9.
2. Perez Teuffer A. Traumatic rupture of the Achilles tendon. Reconstruction by transplant and graft using the lateral peroneus brevis. Orthop Clin North Am 1974;5(1):89–93.
3. Turco VJ, Spinella AJ. Achilles tendon ruptures—peroneus brevis transfer. Foot Ankle 1987;7(4):253–9.
4. Mann RA, Holmes GB, Seale KS, Collins DN. Chronic rupture of the Achilles tendon: a new technique of repair. J Bone Joint Surg 1991;73A(2):214–9.
5. Kann JN, Myerson MS. Surgical management of chronic ruptures of the Achilles tendon. Foot Ankle Clin 1997;2:535–45.
6. Wapner KL, Hecht PJ, Mills RH. Reconstruction of neglected Achilles tendon injury. Orthop Clin North Am 1995;26(2):249–63.
7. Wapner KL, Pavlock GS, Hecht PJ, Naselli F, Walther R. Repair of chronic Achilles tendon rupture with flexor hallucis longus tendon transfer. Foot Ankle 1993;14(8):443–9.
8. Wilcox DK, Bohay DR, Andersen JG. Treatment of chronic Achilles tendon disorders with flexor hallucis longus tendon transfer/augmentation. Foot Ankle Int 2000;21(12):1004–10.
9. Abraham E, Pankovich AM. Neglected rupture of the Achilles tendon. Treatment by V-Y tendinous flap. J Bone Joint Surg 1975;57B(2):253–5.
10. Bosworth DM. Repair of defects in the tendo achillis. J Bone Joint Surg 1956;38A(1):111–4.
11. Jennings AG, Sefton GK. Chronic rupture of tendo Achillis. Long-term results of operative management using polyester tape. J Bone Joint Surg 2002;84B(3):361–3.
12. Dodds WN, Burry HC. The relationship between Achilles tendon rupture and serum uric acid level. Injury 1984;16:94–5.
13. Dent CM, Graham GP. Osteogenesis imperfecta and Achilles tendon rupture. Injury 1991;22:239–40.
14. Arner O, Lindholm A, Orell SR. Histologic changes in subcutaneous rupture of the Achilles tendon. A study of 74 cases. Acta Orthop Scand 1995;116:484–90.
15. Maffulli N, Irwin AS, Kenward MG, Smith F, Porter RW. Achilles tendon rupture and sciatica: a possible correlation. Br J Sports Med 1998;32:174–7.
16. McMaster PE. Tendon and muscle ruptures. Clinical and experimental studies on the causes and location of subcutaneous ruptures. J Bone Joint Surg 1933;15:705–22.
17. Lagergren C, Lindholm A. Vascular distribution in the Achilles tendon. An angiographic and microangiographic study. Acta Orthop Scand 1958;116:491–6.
18. Maffulli N. Current concepts review: rupture of the Achilles tendon. J Bone Joint Surg 1999;81A:1019–36.
19. Kennedy JC, Willis RB. The effects of local steroid injections on tendon: a biomechanical and microscopic correlative study. Am J Sports Med 1976;4:11–21.

20. Royer RJ, Pierfitte C, Netter P. Features of tendon disorders with fluoroquinolones. Therapie 2006;49:75–6.
21. Kannus P, Jozsa L. Histopathological changes preceding spontaneous rupture of a tendon. A controlled study of 891 patients. J Bone Joint Surg 1991;73A(12):1507–25.
22. Valderrabano V, Hintermann B, Csizy M. Anatomic reconstruction of chronic Achilles tendon ruptures. Rational and mid-term results. Am J Sports Med, submitted.
23. Knupp M, Hintermann B. Anatomic repair of the intermediate chronic Achilles tendon rupture. Tech Foot Ankle Surg 2005;4(3):138–42.

11

Treatment of Chronic Achilles Tendon Ruptures with Tendon Transfers

Andrew M. Ebert and Robert B. Anderson

Presentation

Treatment delays after complete rupture of the Achilles tendon are not uncommon, because nearly 20% of patients are misdiagnosed on initial examination.[1] Numerous definitions of what constitutes a "chronic" or late Achilles tendon rupture have been proposed. A functional definition would be those ruptures left untreated for such a time as to prohibit primary tendon repair. Most would agree that this situation will likely be encountered with complete Achilles ruptures beyond the 4 to 6 week mark.[2] Distribution of chronic injuries appears to be equal among males and females, with the average age of presentation between 35 and 60 years. The neglected acute rupture includes the usual history of acute pain or sensation of a "pop" occurring in the calf, with subsequent weakness. However, the subset of patients who sustain recurrent partial ruptures often present with more subtle histories. Those with connective tissue disorders or chronic Achilles tendinosis may relate a long history of intermittent pain and progressive weakness. Gradual lengthening of the musculotendinous unit is mirrored by loss of function. Still other patients may have a history of chronic fluoroquinolone usage, intratendinous cortisone injections, or anabolic steroid abuse.[3,4]

In all cases, patients ultimately present with significant plantarflexion weakness. They usually complain of loss of push-off strength, manifested by difficulty with stair climbing or walking uphill. Asymmetric calf atrophy is the norm. Patients with neglected acute ruptures often have a visible zone of skin depression overlying the separated tendon ends (Fig. 11.1) . However, those with gradual elongation from chronic tendinosis may have generalized thickening of the tendon without a defect. It is important to note that Thompson's squeeze test is often negative when scarring bridges the tendon gaps.

Though the diagnosis of a chronic Achilles tendon injury is often clear from history and examination, imaging studies aid in operative planning. Radiographs may reveal bony avulsions off the calcaneus or proximal retractions of distal tendon calcific deposits. Magnetic resonance imaging (MRI) can quantify the length of tendon retraction; the extent of tendinopathy, fibrosis, and fibrofatty infiltration; and the location of the disruption. All of this information is essential for preoperative planning.[5,6]

J.A. Nunley (ed.), *The Achilles Tendon: Treatment and Rehabilitation*,
DOI: 10.1007/978-1-387-79206-4_11, © Springer Science+Business Media, LLC 2009

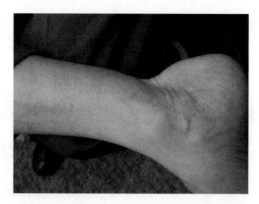

Fig. 11.1. Depressed skin overlying chronic Achilles rupture defect

Treatment

Challenges in treating chronic ruptures of the Achilles tendon are often formidable. Though nonoperative management cannot hope to correct significant loss of function, it may offer some relief to those patients with contraindications to surgery. Patients with known peripheral vascular disease, active infections, poorly controlled systemic diseases (e.g., rheumatoid arthritis), and the low-demand elderly can be treated nonoperatively. Skin disease or scarring from previous injuries or surgery should likewise be considered before surgical planning. In these cases, conservative modalities, including bracing, casting, and therapy, may offer the patient the best option in view of the risks entailed with surgery.[6,7] Bracing, however, cannot rectify a calcaneal gait from an overlengthened Achilles tendon since extreme ankle dorsiflexion is difficult to block with a brace that does not also eliminate plantar flexion.

Most patients with significant functional compromise from chronic Achilles ruptures are best treated surgically. The surgical technique employed is dictated by a number of key principles. Both the gap between tendon ends and the condition of the remaining gastroc-soleus musculature must be considered. In cases in which the gap or diseased Achilles measures less than 6 cm and the gastrocnemius muscle has not suffered undue atrophy, advancement procedures are helpful and avoid the need for tendon transfers. The goal is to "span the gap" (see discussion of advancement techniques in Chapter 10).

Tendon Transfers

Long-standing ruptures with significant muscle atrophy and tendon retraction often require tendon transfers. When the gap or diseased Achilles measures greater than 6 cm or poor muscle exists proximally, a tendon transfer is recommended not only to restore function but also to span the defect with viable tissue.

Tendon transfers have been long described in the treatment of both acute and chronic Achilles rupture. The variety of described transfer techniques is remarkable. Coughlin[8] notes that in 1931 Platt[9] described the use of the posterior tibial tendon to augment Achilles repairs. With the evolution of less compromising transfers, this technique has fallen out of favor. A number of authors have explored the use of plantaris muscle tendon transfers for Achilles ruptures.[10,11] Because it may be bound in scar tissue or be altogether absent, as well as due to its small size, it is not considered a good transfer option for chronic Achilles ruptures.

Peroneus Brevis Transfer

Previous reports by other physicians led Turco and Spinella[12] to describe the use of the peroneus brevis tendon, which is routed through the calcaneus. After identifying and detaching the tendon from its insertion on the base of the fifth metatarsal, they passed the peroneus brevis tendon through a lateral to medial calcaneal drill hole. The tendon was then sutured to the Achilles so that it spanned the rupture site (Fig. 11.2) . The authors' report included a mix of 40 acute, chronic, and recurrent Achilles ruptures with apparently good results. Sacrificing the peroneus brevis, however, compromises foot eversion and lateral ankle stability, and the repair fails to act "in phase" with foot plantar flexors.

Flexor Digitorum Longus Transfer

In 1991, Mann et al.[13] described using the flexor digitorum longus (FDL) tendon transfer for chronic Achilles ruptures. The Achilles is approached from a posteromedial incision, and interposed fibrotic tissue is debrided from between the Achilles tendon ends. A second incision on the medial border of the foot allows for harvest of the FDL tendon just proximal to its divisions at the knot of Henry. The distal FDL tendon stump is sutured to the adjacent flexor hallucis longus (FHL) while maintaining the lesser toe interphalangeal (IP) joints in neutral extension. The proximal FDL tendon is pulled into the proximal posterior medial ankle incision behind the neurovascular bundle. It is then passed through a medial to lateral calcaneal drill hole and sutured to itself. The authors reported good to excellent results in six of seven patients treated with this technique. They had no lesser toe sequelae from harvest of the FDL.

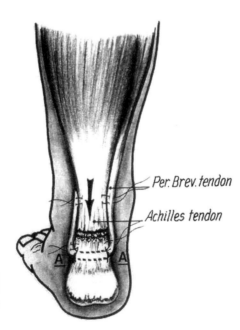

Per. Brev. tendon

Achilles tendon

Fig. 11.2. Peroneus brevis transfer and weave. (From Turco and Spinella,[12] with permission of Wolters Kluwer Health.)

Flexor Hallucis Longus Transfer

Popularized by Wapner et al.,[14,15] the FHL is currently the workhorse of tendon transfers for chronic Achilles ruptures. This transfer has proved reliable in multiple studies and has several advantages over other tendon transfer techniques. As highlighted by Silver et al.,[16] the plantarflexion strength of the FHL is second only to the gastroc-soleus complex. By comparison, the FDL plantarflexion strength is 50% that of the FHL while the peroneus brevis is approximately 70%. The FHL contractile force is more closely aligned with that of the Achilles and acts in phase with the native gastroc-soleus complex. It avoids the functional mismatch of substituting an evertor for a plantar flexor as seen with the peroneus brevis transfer. While the sacrifice of a major foot evertor may prove problematic with peroneus brevis transfer, patients rarely perceive any loss of hallux flexion strength with FHL sacrifice.[17]

The FHL can be harvested through a separate incision on the plantar or medial surface of the foot or from the same posteromedial ankle incision that is used to approach the ruptured Achilles tendon. Cadaveric studies have demonstrated that the distal harvest from the foot yields an additional 10 to 12 cm of tendon, which may prove useful in cases of significant Achilles loss with poor tendon remnants. This extra tendon can be woven through the remaining portions of the Achilles tendon as a tendon substitute, thus spanning the gap as well as functioning as an active tendon transfer. Often, however, advancement procedures may allow for a secure tendon repair. Because of gastroc-soleus muscle atrophy, however, the surgeon may feel the need to augment plantarflexion strength. In such cases, the morbidity of a second incision can be avoided and the FHL can be harvested from the same postero-medial approach and then inserted into the calcaneus.

The classic two-incision FHL transfer is performed with the patient prone (Fig. 11.3) . A medial midfoot incision is made along the inferior border of the first metatarsal and the abductor muscle is reflected plantar. The FHL and FDL tendons are identified, and they are then tenodesed as far distally as possible with the toes in neutral flexion. The FHL is next transected and any intertendonous FDL–FHL connections must be released (Fig. 11.4) . The second incision is made posteromedially at the ankle along the medial border of the Achilles. The Achilles tendon ends are identified, and any interposed fibrosis is debrided back to healthy tendon ends. The fascia of the posterior compartment is opened, and the cut FHL tendon is pulled into the operative field. Intersecting superior and medial drill holes are made in the calcaneus, and the FHL tendon is then passed through this bone tunnel. The tendon can then be sutured back on itself or woven through the Achilles remnant (Fig. 11.5) . The tendon should be tensioned maximally with the foot in 15 degrees of plantarflexion. Prepping the contralateral extremity allows for intraoperative tension comparison between the two feet. When compared, the reconstructed side should be equal to, or slightly more than, resting equinus. Postoperatively, the foot is immobilized in plantarflexion for 4 weeks and the patient kept non–weight bearing. A short leg walking cast is then placed for an additional 4 weeks. Range of motion and strengthening exercises with a heel lift are started at 8 weeks. Aggressive exercise is prohibited until the 6-month mark.

The FHL harvest/transfer can also be performed through a single postero-medial incision.[17–19] The fascia overlying the deep posterior compartment is incised longitudinally, and the FHL tendon is identified (Fig. 11.6) . The tendon

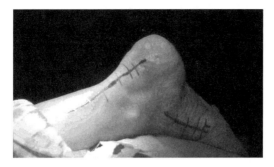

Fig. 11.3. Positioning and incisions for two-incision flexor hallucis longus (FHL) transfer

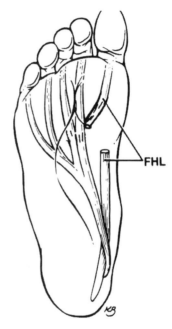

Fig. 11.4. Artist's depiction of FHL harvest and tenodesis of distal stump with flexor digitorum longus (FDL). (From Wapner et al.,[14] with permission of Wolters Kluwer Health.)

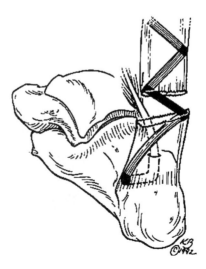

Fig. 11.5. The flexor hallucis longus tendon is routed through interconnecting superior and medial tunnels through the calcaneus. The tendon is then woven through the Achilles and can be used to span a gap between tendon stumps. (From Wapner et al.,[14] with permission of Wolters Kluwer Health.)

is harvested as distally as possible as it courses under the sustentaculum (Fig. 11.7) ; the ankle, foot, and great toe are in maximum plantarflexion. The tendon should by transected in a direction away from the nearby neurovascular bundle. The FHL tendon is secured with a grasping suture; next, a drill bit is chosen of appropriate diameter to create a bony tunnel to allow for tendon passage (Fig. 11.8) . The calcaneal bone tunnel is created approximately 2 to 3 cm anterior to the native Achilles insertion (Fig. 11.9) . A suture passer or long Keith needle is then used to pass the FHL grasping suture arms through a small stab wound in the plantar aspect of the heel. The FHL tendon is then pulled plantar through the bone tunnel and anchored with an interference screw under moderate tension while maintaining the foot in approximately 15 to 20 degrees of plantar flexion (Fig. 11.10) . The transferred FHL can also be sutured to the remaining Achilles in a side-to-side fashion (Fig. 11.11). Incisions are closed in a standard fashion followed by application of a well-padded, short, leg splint maintaining the foot in 20 to 30 degrees of plantarflexion. A drain is not routinely used.

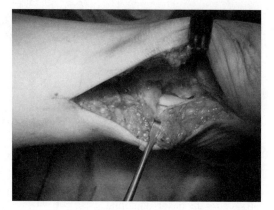

Fig. 11.6. Single-incision FHL harvest and transfer. FHL tendon is identified in the posterior compartment

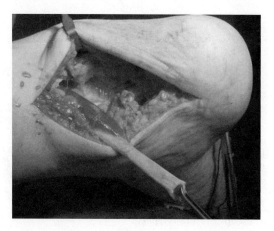

Fig. 11.7. Tendon is harvested as far distally as possible, taking care to protect nearby neurovascular structures

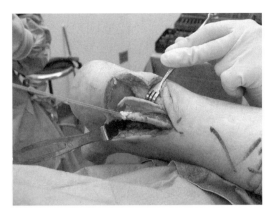

Fig. 11.8. Tendon is secured with a grasping stitch for passage through bone tunnel

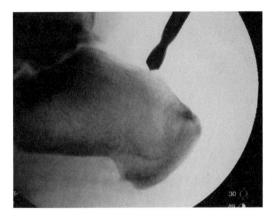

Fig. 11.9. Bone tunnel is created anterior to Achilles insertion

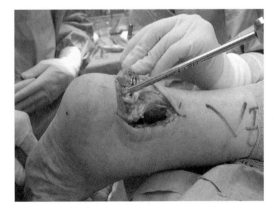

Fig. 11.10. Tendon is passed and secured with a bioabsorbable interference screw

The patient is kept non–weightbearing for the first 2 weeks. At the 2-week mark, the patient's leg may be placed in a walker boot with 20 degrees of plantarflexion. Active range-of-motion exercises out of the boot are encouraged

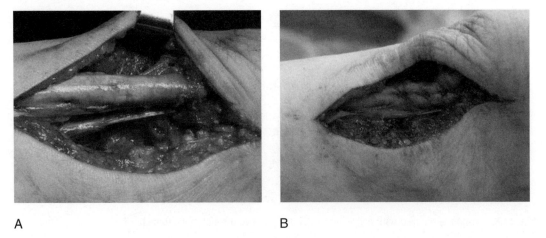

A   B

Fig. 11.11. (A,B) Transferred FHL and Achilles are sutured together, completing the reconstruction

at this time. At 4 weeks postoperatively, full weight bearing is begun in a walker boot with a heel lift. The heel lift height is gradually decreased over the ensuing 4 weeks, and therapy is begun for strengthening and motion.

Good results for FHL transfers for chronic Achilles tendon disorders have been documented in several studies. At average follow-up of 17 months (range, 3 to 30), Wapner et al.[14] reported good to excellent results in six of seven patients with chronic ruptures treated with FHL transfer. Den Hartog[19] documented good to excellent results in 23 of 26 patients who underwent FHL transfer through a single posteromedial incision for chronic Achilles tendinosis. Similarly, Wilcox et al.[20] evaluated 20 patients (mean age 61) who underwent FHL transfer for treatment of chronic Achilles tendinopathy at a mean of 14 months following surgery, and found that 90% of patients scored 70 or higher on the AOFAS scale.[20] Despite some residual plantarflexion strength deficits, most patients are highly satisfied with the functional improvement they gain from the FHL transfer, as in the following case study.

Case Study

A 48-year-old teacher sustained an ankle injury while hiking outdoors. He felt a pop that was followed by pain and swelling. He was seen at the emergency room of a local hospital, where he was told he had sprained his ankle. He was placed in a stirrup-type ankle brace and told to follow up with his primary care provider. At 5 months postinjury, he continued to complain of persistent weakness and difficulty with stair climbing despite physical therapy. An MRI was obtained by his primary care physician, which demonstrated fibrosis and edema in the Achilles tendon consistent with a neglected rupture.

At the time of presentation, examination demonstrated significant calf atrophy on the affected extremity and a palpable gap in the Achilles tendon. Because of his continued weakness, he was offered reconstruction. Intraoperative examination of the tendon demonstated a 6-cm zone of fibrosis between the ends of the native tendon. This was excised. His native gastrocnemius-soleus complex was noted to be quite atrophied. With these factors in mind, a decision was made to perform an FHL transfer with distal harvest to optimize tendon length. The FHL tendon was tenotomized just distal to the metatarsophalangeal (MTP) joint (Fig. 11.12) .

Intratendonous connections between the FHL and FDL were released at the knot of Henry in the plantar midfoot (Fig. 11.13) . The tendon was delivered and passed through intersecting calcaneal drill holes (Fig. 11.14) . A tendon weaver was used to pass the FHL through the native Achilles and to bridge the intervening gap (Fig. 11.15) .

The patient had an uneventful postoperative period. He began physical therapy at 8 weeks postsurgery for strengthening and motion. By 12 months postsurgery, he had returned to all normal activities with no complaints of weakness.

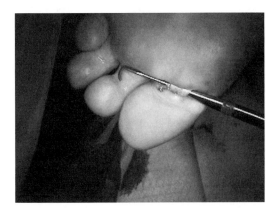

Fig. 11.12. Distal harvest of FHL tendon through small stab incision for maximal tendon length. In this technique, tenodesis of the distal FHL stump to the FDL is not performed

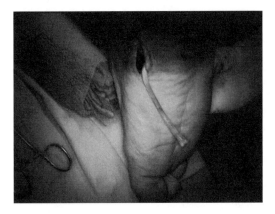

Fig. 11.13. Tendon must mobilized at the knot of Henry, where it often tethered to surrounding soft tissue

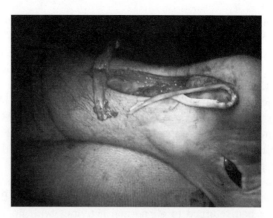

Fig. 11.14. The FHL is delivered and passed though a calcaneal bone tunnel

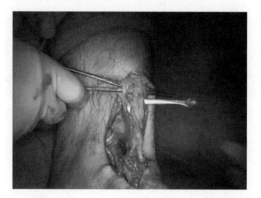

Fig. 11.15. Tendon is weaved through native Achilles stumps, completing the reconstruction

References

1. Maffulli N. Rupture of the Achilles tendon. J Bone Joint Surg 1999;81A:1019–36.
2. Gabel S, Manoli A. Foot fellow's review: neglected rupture of the Achilles tendon. Foot Ankle Int 1994;15:512–7.
3. McGarvey W, Singh D, Trevino S. Partial Achilles tendon ruptures associated with fluoroquinolone antibiotics: a case report and literature review. Foot Ankle Int 1996;17:496–8.
4. Laseter JT, Russell JA. Anabolic steroid-induced tendon pathology: a review of the literature. Med Sci Sports Exerc 1991;23(1):1–3.
5. Deutsch AL, Lund PJ, Mink JH. MR imaging and diagnostic ultrasound in the evaluation of Achilles tendon disorders, Foot Ankle Clin 1997;2:391.
6. Carden DG, Noble J, Chalmers J, et al. Rupture of the calcaneal tendon; the early and late management. J Bone Joint Surg Br 1987;69:416.
7. Cetti R, Christensen SE, Ejsted R, et al. Operative versus nonoperative treatment of Achilles tendon rupture: a prospective randomized study and review of the literature. Am J Sports Med 1993;21:791.
8. Coughlin MJ. Disorders of tendons. In: Coughlin MJ, Mann RA, eds. Surgery of the Foot and Ankle, 7th ed. St Louis: Mosby, 1999:844–50.
9. Platt H. Observations on some tendon ruptures, Br Med J 1931;1:611–5.

10. Lynn T. Repair of the torn Achilles tendon using the plantaris tendon as a reinforcing membrane. J Bone Joint Surg 1966;48A:268–72.

11. Schedl R, Fasol P. Achilles tendon repair with plantaris tendon compared with repair using polyglycol threads. J Trauma 1979;19:189–94.

12. Turco VJ, Spinella AJ. Achilles tendon ruptures—peroneus brevis transfer. Foot Ankle 1987;7(4):253–9.

13. Mann R, Holmes G, Seale K, Collins D. Chronic rupture of the Achilles tendon: a new technique of repair, J Bone Joint Surg 1991;73A:214–9.

14. Wapner LK, Pavlock GS, Hecht PJ, et al. Repair of chronic Achilles tendon rupture with flexor hallucis longus tendon transfer. Foot Ankle 1993;14:443–9.

15. Wapner KL, Hecht PJ, Mills RH Jr. Reconstruction of neglected Achilles tendon injury. Orthop Clin North Am 1995;26(2):249–63.

16. Silver R, de la Garza J, Rang M. The myth of muscle balance: a study of relative strengths and excursions of normal muscles about the foot and ankle. J Bone Joint Surg 1985;67B:432–7.

17. Coull R, Flavin R, Stevens MM. Flexor hallucis longus tendon transfer: evaluation of postoperative morbidity. Foot Ankle Int 2003;24(12):931–4.

18. Hansen S. Trauma to the heel cord. In: Jahss M, ed. Disorders of the Foot and Ankle: Medical and Surgical Management, 2nd ed. Philadelphia: WB Saunders, 1991:2355–60.

19. Den Hartog BD. Flexor hallucis longus transfer for chronic Achilles tendonosis. Foot Ankle Int 2003;24(3):233–7.

20. Wilcox DK, Bohay DR, Anderson JG. Treatment of chronic Achilles tendon disorders with FHL tendon transfer/augmentation. Foot Ankle Int 2000;21(12):1004–10.

12

Free Tissue Reconstruction

Kurtis Moyer and L. Scott Levin

Reconstruction of the Achilles tendon in the face of skin deficiency is a difficult surgical dilemma. Acute rupture with extensive local soft tissue trauma, as well as chronic rupture with or without associated infection, requires a more sophisticated reconstruction.

The reconstructive algorithm for an Achilles tendon rupture is well documented in the literature. Small segmental tendon defects, less than 2 cm without soft tissue trauma, can usually be primarily repaired with good success.[1] Larger tendon defects have been successfully reconstructed with V-Y tendon flaps, gastrocnemius turn-down flaps, fascia lata grafts, Marlex mesh, and flexor hallucis longus interposition grafts.[1–5] All of these repairs rely on the presence of an adequate soft tissue envelope to allow wound closure, which is critical for proper tendon excursion, protection of the tendon from desiccation, and durability during ambulation. In the face of significant soft tissue loss associated with an Achilles tendon injury, such methods are unable to provide a functional Achilles tendon restoration.

Absence of an adequate soft tissue envelope adjacent to the Achilles tendon can result from trauma, but can also occur due to complications associated with patient comorbidities, such as diabetes.[6] Acute ruptures that are primarily repaired may become infected, resulting in significant soft tissue loss after debridement with exposure of the Achilles tendon. Likewise a recurrent rupture of a previously repaired Achilles tendon can compromise the soft tissue envelope, preventing wound closure over a subsequent tendon repair. In addition, patient comorbidities such as diabetes, venous insufficiency, and peripheral vascular disease can often lead to poor wound healing, incisional dehiscence, and exposure of the Achilles tendon. Poor wound healing usually requires the transplantation of well-vascularized soft tissue to adequately protect the Achilles tendon repair. Due to the lack of adequate adjacent tissue available, such as a local flap, reconstruction of both the tendon and soft tissue requires a more sophisticated repair.

Complex Achilles tendon injuries include two elements that need to be reconstructed. There is a need to repair the tendon or provide a suitable graft to restore functional continuity. In addition to tendon repair, there is a need for skin and soft tissue to create an adequate environment for tendon excursion.

J.A. Nunley (ed.), *The Achilles Tendon: Treatment and Rehabilitation*,
DOI: 10.1007/978-1-387-79206-4_12, © Springer Science+Business Media, LLC 2009

The goals of complex Achilles tendon reconstruction, therefore, may demand a composite reconstruction of both of these components. Although one or both of these elements may be reconstructed using individual components, such as a Marlex mesh or tensor fascia lata graft for tendon continuity followed by soft tissue transposition for coverage, the ability to perform free tissue transfer through microsurgical techniques allows for a single-stage composite flap reconstruction.[5–11]

Free tissue transfer through microsurgical techniques has advanced the state of Achilles reconstruction. Since the first reported cases of tissue transfer for lower extremity reconstruction in the 1970s, significant advances have been made in the understanding of the microvascular architecture of free flaps.[12,13] This is due in large part to Taylor's[13–15] work to define angiosomes. The description of composite flaps that contain different tissue components enables reconstructive surgeons to adhere to Sir Harold Gillie's principle of replacing "like with like."[16] Free tissue transfer allows the surgeon to transplant tendon, fascia, skin, soft tissue, muscle, and bone all within a single vascularized unit or composite flap. The use of vascularized tissue through microsurgical techniques has been documented to decrease the rate of wound infections, and improve wound healing.[17–19] The thickness of a flap can also be selected, allowing for better contour and cosmetic appeal. Resurfacing of the Achilles tendon requires thin flaps that are durable and allow for normal shoe wear.

Patient Evaluation

The first step in Achilles reconstruction involves determining the components needed for reconstruction. Components are dependent on the tendon's functional status prior to repair. Often the extent of the defect is not realized until debridement is completed. Extensive removal of all devitalized tissue is essential to ensure a successful reconstruction. After debridement has been completed, the wound is assessed to determine what is required for reconstruction.

Patient evaluation prior to reconstructions entails a thorough lower extremity vascular examination, including palpating the dorsalis pedis and posterior tibial pulses, as well as performing an ankle-to-brachial index (ABI). Findings that reveal absent distal pulses or a diminished ABI indicate the need for further vascular studies, such as an angiogram. Essential to a successful microsurgical reconstruction is access to adequate recipient arterial and venous conduits for the microsurgical anastomosis. In preparation for microsurgical reconstruction, the finding of significant inflow or outflow disease ultimately requires an intervention to reestablish perfusion. Depending on the nature and location of the occlusion, this may include the use of a stent or formal bypass grafting prior to, or at the same time as, the reconstruction. Once the patient has an adequate vascular supply to the lower extremity, the process of flap selection occurs.

Flap Selection

The authors' preferred method of reconstructing Achilles tendon defects is the radial forearm flap (see Case Studies 1 and 2, below). The radial forearm flap was described in the 1980s and is an excellent choice for Achilles tendon composite reconstructions.[20–22] The flap has the capability of including skin, soft tissue, fascia, palmaris longus tendon, and a portion of the radius all on a single vascular pedicle.

The radial forearm flap is a fasciocutaneous flap based on the radial artery. Prior to dissection of this flap, the patient needs to have an Allen's test performed in order to document a patent palmar arch. The cutaneous skin paddle can be as large as 10 × 20 cm or two-thirds the size of the forearm, allowing for coverage of a significant soft tissue defect.[16] Included within this flap are the palmaris longus tendon and its associated paratenon. The inclusion of the palmaris tendon with its paratenon ensures adequate tendon glide for a functional dynamic repair when incorporated for segmental Achilles tendon defects. If a sensate flap is desired, the lateral antebrachial nerve can also be included.

The radial forearm free flap is thin, yet durable, making it an excellent choice for resurfacing of the Achilles tendon region. The radial artery is infrequently affected by atherosclerosis, making it a good choice in patients with a history of peripheral vascular disease.

A skin graft is often required for donor site closure (Fig. 12.1). The palmaris longus tendon is absent in about 10% of the population; however, there have been reports of incorporating the brachioradialis tendon within the flap, which has also yielded good success. The flap is not usable in patients who lack a patent deep and superficial arch system in the hand.

Case Study 1

A 69-year-old woman with no significant medical history suffered an acute Achilles tendon rupture that was repaired primarily. The patient subsequently developed a soft tissue infection and draining sinus overlying the tendon repair. An early attempt at debridement and split-thickness graft coverage resulted in further wound breakdown, infection, and exposure of the Achilles tendon repair. Figure 12.2 demonstrates exposure of the suture repair with an area of soft tissue infection. The area was debrided sharply and treated with local wound care in preparation for coverage. The defect required soft tissue and a tendon interposition graft for a 4 cm segmental defect in the Achilles tendon. Physical exam revealed palpable dorsalis pedis and posterior tibial artery pulses. Figure 12.3 shows the preoperative markings of the radial forearm

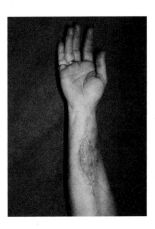

Fig. 12.1. Radial forearm flap donor site with split-thickness skin graft

Fig. 12.2. Wound breakdown with exposure of previous Achilles tendon repair and split-thickness skin graft coverage

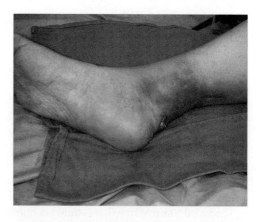

Fig. 12.3. Radial forearm flap design with palmaris longus (P.L.) tendon inclusion

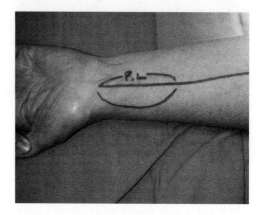

flap and the associated palmaris longus tendon. The radial forearm flap was anastomosed to the posterior tibial artery and is shown in the flap inset in Figure 12.4. The patient remained non–weight bearing and in a posterior splint for 6 weeks with subsequent incremental increase in weight transfer. Within 3 months the patient had a full range of dorsiflexion and plantarflexion, as well as full weight-bearing capabilities.

Case Study 2

A 57-year-old man had a history of diabetes and peripheral vascular disease. A previous lower extremity bypass procedure on the involved extremity had been performed with a saphenous vein graft from the same leg. The patient suffered an Achilles tendon rupture of his left leg that was primarily repaired and the soft tissue closed directly. Subsequently, the patient developed a wound infection leading to the destruction of local soft tissue. The Achilles tendon repair was intact and the tendon was viable. The wound, as well as the scar from the previous saphenous vein harvest, are shown in Figure 12.5. A physical examination showed that the patient had palpable dorsalis pedis and posterior tibial pulses and an ABI of 1.0. The wound was debrided, resulting in a skin defect and an exposed Achilles tendon with intact repair. The flap was harvested as a fasciocutaneous flap on the radial artery and anastomosed

Fig. 12.4. Radial forearm flap inset with complete coverage of wound

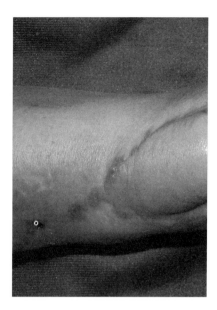

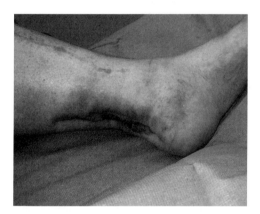

Fig. 12.5. Wound breakdown of previous Achilles tendon repair after infection

to the posterior tibial artery. Insetting of the flap with complete soft tissue coverage of the Achilles tendon is shown in Figure 12.6. The patient was again in a posterior splint and non–weight bearing for 6 weeks. By 3 months, he was full weight bearing with full plantar- and dorsiflexion range of motion.

Although the radial forearm flap remains the authors' preferred method for Achilles tendon reconstruction, there are additional flaps that are used when the radial forearm flap is not available. Reasons for the inability to use the forearm flap include trauma to the upper arm with damage to the vascular supply of the flap. Lack of a patent superficial and deep palmar arch or a patient's request not to have a large scar on the volar aspect of the forearm are additional reasons not to use the radial forearm flap. The authors prefer to use a lateral arm or scapular flap in these settings, depending on the patient's body habitus (see Case Study 3, below).

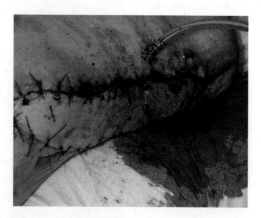

Fig. 12.6. Radial forearm flap inset with complete coverage of wound

The lateral arm flap was also described in the 1980s.[6,9,22] Like the radial forearm flap, it can be harvested as a fasciocutaneous flap with associated humeral osseous segment and sensitized through the posterior antebrachial cutaneous nerve. The flap is based on the posterior radial collateral artery and can be harvested with the triceps tendon. The pedicle is capable of sustaining a cutaneous paddle of 6 cm in length and 12 cm long.[16]

Benefits of the flap include the ability to take a composite flap with the previously mentioned components. Like the radial forearm flap, the lateral arm flap is thin and durable; but unlike the radial forearm flap, its donor defect can be primarily closed if the width of the cutaneous paddle is less than 6 cm, resulting in improved cosmesis.

Morbidity of the flap includes numbness of the upper lateral forearm secondary to the harvesting of the posterior antebrachial cutaneous nerve. A small vascular pedicle, often 1 mm in diameter, can increase the difficulty level of the anastomosis. Increased flap bulk in patients with a large body habitus may necessitate flap debulking at a later stage. An example of a when a lateral arm flap could be used for reconstruction is demonstrated in the following case study.

Case Study 3

A 51-year-old man suffered a traumatic degloving injury to the soft tissue envelope of the left Achilles region. The tendon was intact and immediate coverage was attempted with a split-thickness skin graft. The patient was otherwise healthy with no comorbidities. The patient subsequently developed a soft tissue infection with exposure of the underlying Achilles tendon. Local wound care was attempted without success. The defect is shown in Figure 12.7. An examination revealed that the patient had a palpable dorsalis pedis and posterior tibial artery pulse. After operative debridement, the resulting defect is shown in Figure 12.8. A lateral arm flap was selected secondary to the patient's preference not to have a donor scar on his forearm. The lateral arm flap offered a reasonable alternative due to the patient's thin body habitus.

Fig. 12.7. Wound breakdown after Achilles tendon repair and split-thickness skin graft coverage

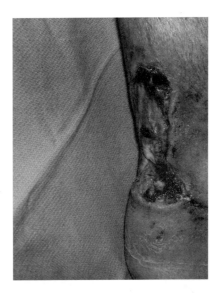

Fig. 12.8. Achilles wound after surgical debridement

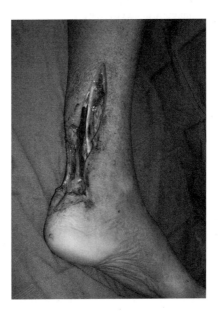

Figure 12.9 demonstrates the operative flap design and the flap insetting (Fig. 12.10). The patient followed our standard protocol of non–weight bearing for 6 weeks, and return to progressive weight bearing and ambulation within 3 months.

The scapular flap (see Case Study 4, below) is another option when attempting to reconstruct an Achilles tendon injury.[23–25]The flap is based on the circumflex scapular artery, which is a branch of the subscapular artery. The flap can include components of skin, soft tissue, and an osseous portion of the scapula. The skin paddle can be up to 20 cm long and 10 cm wide.[16] Unlike the previous two flaps, it is not a sensate flap and does not include a tendon.

Fig. 12.9. Lateral arm flap design

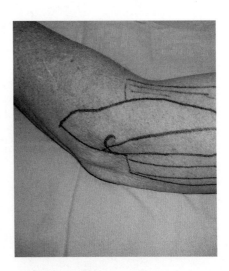

Fig. 12.10. Lateral arm flap inset with complete wound coverage

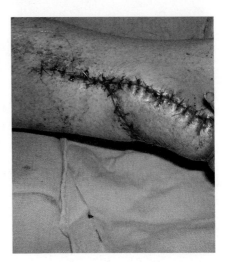

This flap offers the ability to primarily close the defect if the width of the flap is kept under 10 cm. The vascular pedicle is large in diameter, facilitating the microsurgical anastomosis. The morbidity of the donor site is low.

A disadvantage includes the need for a lateral decubitus position in order to facilitate harvesting of the flap. Another disadvantage is the inability to include a sensory nerve in the flap, as well as the flap being too bulky in an individual with a large body habitus.

Case Study 4

A 47-year-old woman suffered a traumatic injury to the soft tissue envelope surrounding the Achilles tendon region with an intact tendon. Treating the region with local wound care, and the patient present for definitive coverage, proved unsuccessful. The patient was otherwise healthy and had a palpable dorsalis pedis and posterior tibial artery signal. Figure 12.11 shows the insetting of the scapular flap and the patient plantar flexing at 3 months after surgery (Fig. 12.12).

The previously listed flaps are those that the authors routinely use for reconstruction of Achilles tendon defects. There are, however, many other flap options in the armamentarium of the reconstructive surgeon. The literature cites the use of the anterior lateral thigh flap, which is based on the lateral femoral circumflex vessels as a fasciocutaneous flap that can be harvested with tensor fascia lata and used to repair segmental Achilles tendon defects.[26,27] In addition, the literature supports the use of a composite groin flap based on the superior circumflex iliac artery.[28] The components of this flap provide not only a soft tissue envelope, but also an osseous segment of iliac crest and external oblique fascia that can be rolled to form an interposition graft for large Achilles tendon defects. Others have reported success with using the

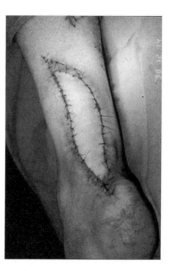

Fig. 12.11. Scapular flap inset with complete wound coverage

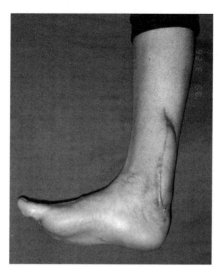

Fig. 12.12. Plantar flexion 3 months after scapular flap coverage of Achilles wound

latissimus myocutaneous flap as a single-stage procedure for reconstruction of large segmental tendon defects.[29]

Conclusion

Many of the composite flaps for microsurgical reconstruction have been mentioned here, but this list is certainly not exhaustive. Achilles tendon injuries are often repaired successfully through primary repair and reapproximation of the soft tissues. However, with associated trauma and localized soft tissue destruction, the task of reconstruction becomes a formidable one. Although a role for local flaps is not acknowledged, there are significant limitations to the use of these local flaps, especially in the trauma patient. Microsurgical techniques enable transferring composite flaps with all of the needed elements for reconstruction, eliminating the need for allografts and mesh, which increase the rates of infection and scar formation, leading to lack of tendon excursion and soft tissue loss. The advent of microsurgical techniques gives the reconstructive surgeon options to solve these complex problems.

References

1. Leppilahti J, Orava S. Total Achilles tendon rupture. A review. Sports Med 1998;25(2):79–100.
2. Choksey A, Soonawalla D, Murray J. Repair of neglected Achilles tendon ruptures with Marlex mesh. Injury 1996;27(3):215–7.
3. Nistor L. Surgical and non-surgical treatment of Achilles tendon rupture. A prospective randomized study. J Bone Joint Surg [Am] 1981;63(3):394–9.
4. Ozaki J, Fujiki J, Sugimoto K, et al. Reconstruction of neglected Achilles tendon rupture with Marlex mesh. Clin Orthop Rel Res 1989(238):204–8.
5. Wapner KL, Hecht PJ, Mills RH. Reconstruction of neglected Achilles tendon injury. Orthop Clin North Am 1995;26(2):249–63.
6. Ronel DN, . Recent advances in the reconstruction of complex Achilles tendon defects. Microsurgery 2004;24(1):18–23.
7. Berthe JV, Toussaint D, Coessens BC. One-stage reconstruction of an infected skin and Achilles tendon defect with a composite distally planned lateral arm flap. Plast Reconstr Surg 1998;102(5):1618–22.
8. Dabernig J, Shilov B, Schumacher O, . Functional reconstruction of Achilles tendon defects combined with overlaying skin defects using a free tensor fasciae latae flap. J Plast Reconstr Aesthet Surg 2006;59(2):142–7.
9. Haas F, Seibert FJ, Koch H, . Reconstruction of combined defects of the Achilles tendon and the overlying soft tissue with a fascia lata graft and a free fasciocutaneous lateral arm flap. Ann Plast Surg 2003;51(4):376–82.
10. Hallock GG. Free-flap coverage of the exposed Achilles tendon. Plast Reconstr Surg 1989;83(4):710–6.
11. Papp C, Todoroff BP, Windhofer C, . Partial and complete reconstruction of Achilles tendon defects with the fasciocutaneous infragluteal free flap. Plast Reconstr Surg 2003;112(3):777–83.
12. Antia NH, Buch VI. Transfer of an abdominal dermo-fat graft by direct anastomosis of blood vessels. Br J Plast Surg 1971;24(1):15–9.
13. Daniel RK, Taylor GI. Distant transfer of an island flap by microvascular anastomoses. A clinical technique. Plast Reconstr Surg 1973;52(2):111–7.
14. Taylor GI. The angiosomes of the body and their supply to perforator flaps. Clin Plast Surg 2003;30(3):331–42, v.

15. Taylor GI, Palmer JH. The vascular territories (angiosomes) of the body: experimental study and clinical applications. Br J Plast Surg 1987;40(2):113–41.
16. Serafin D. Atlas of Microsurgical Composite Tissue Transplantation, 1st ed. Philadelphia: WB Saunders, 1996.
17. Calderon W, Chang N, Mathes SJ, . Comparison of the effect of bacterial inoculation in musculocutaneous and fasciocutaneous flaps. Plast Reconstr Surg 1986;77(5):785–94.
18. Chang N, Mathes SJ. Comparison of the effect of bacterial inoculation in musculocutaneous and random-pattern flaps. Plast Reconstr Surg 1982;70(1):1–10.
19. Gosain A, Chang N, Mathes SJ, . A study of the relationship between blood flow and bacterial inoculation in musculocutaneous and fasciocutaneous flaps. Plast Reconstr Surg 1990;86(6):1152–62; discussion 1163.
20. Chun JK, Margoles, SL, and Birnbaum, JW. Radial forearm free flap for salvage of Achilles-tendon repair wounds. J Reconstr Microsurg 2000;16(7):519–23.
21. Stanec S, Stanec Z, Delimar D, . A composite forearm free flap for the secondary repair of the ruptured Achilles tendon. Plast Reconstr Surg 1999;104(5):1409–12.
22. Waris TH, Kaarela OI, Raatikainen TK, . Microvascular flaps from the lateral arm and radial forearm for the repair of defects of the Achilles tendon region. Case report. Scand J Plast Reconstr Surg Hand Surg 1991;25(1):87–9.
23. Monsivais JL, PA Nitz, TJ Scully. The free cutaneous scapular flap in lower extremity reconstruction. Mil Med 1987;152(5):255–9.
24. Koshima I, Soeda S. Repair of a wide defect of the lower leg with the combined scapular and parascapular flap. Br J Plast Surg 1985;38(4):518–21.
25. Gilbert A, Teot L. The free scapular flap. Plast Reconstr Surg 1982;69(4):601–4.
26. Lee JW, Yu JC, Shieh SJ, . Reconstruction of the Achilles tendon and overlying soft tissue using antero-lateral thigh free flap. Br J Plast Surg 2000;53(7):574–7.
27. Lin CH, Wei FC, Lin YT, . Lateral circumflex femoral artery system: warehouse for functional composite free-tissue reconstruction of the lower leg. J Trauma 2006;60(5):1032–6.
28. Coskunfirat OK, Sheu TJ, Jeng SF, . Reconstruction of Achilles tendon and overlying skin with composite groin-fascial free flap: a case report of 14-year follow-up. Plast Reconstr Surg 2003;112(1):215–9.
29. Lee HB, Lew DH, Oh SH, . Simultaneous reconstruction of the Achilles tendon and soft-tissue defect using only a latissimus dorsi muscle free flap. Plast Reconstr Surg 1999;104(1):111–9.

Section IV

Achilles Tendinopathy

13

Noninsertional Achilles Tendinopathy: An Overview

Mark E. Easley and Ian L.D. Le

As our society becomes increasingly more health conscious, participation in both competitive and recreational sports activities continues to see unprecedented growth. Consequently, there is a continued rise in the prevalence of sports overuse injuries. Tendon injuries account for 30% to 50% of all injures related to sports, and Achilles tendon disorders account for a substantial proportion of these injuries.[1] Achilles injuries occur annually in 7% to 9% of athletes participating in running, basketball, volleyball, and squash.[2,3] The physicians treating these athletes must have a sound understanding of noninsertional Achilles pathology to minimize morbidity and enable patients to return to their desired level of activity in a timely manner without residual or recurrent pain.

This chapter focuses on the terminology, relevant anatomy, epidemiology, and pathophysiology that provide a foundation for proper diagnosis and treatment of noninsertional Achilles tendinopathy.

Terminology

Achilles tendinopathy is a broad term that can be applied to any disorder afflicting the Achilles tendon. More specifically, Clain and Baxter[4] categorized Achilles tendinopathy as insertional and noninsertional, a distinction that must be made because the two conditions are distinct disorders with different underlying pathophysiologies and treatment options.

The historic nomenclature pertaining to noninsertional disorders of the Achilles tendon has led to confusion among health care providers. Numerous terms have been cited in the medical literature in reference to noninsertional disorders including *Achillodynia, tendopathy, tendinosis, partial rupture, paratendonitis, tenosynovitis, tendovaginitis,* and *peritendinitis.* Furthermore, terms such as *Achilles tendonitis* and *tendinitis* inaccurately imply an underlying inflammatory condition, despite the histologic absence of inflammatory cells and mediators in chronic noninsertional Achilles tendinopathy. Maffulli's group[5,6] emphasized the distinction between a clinical and histopathologic diagnosis and assigned the term *Achilles tendinopathy* to the clinical constellation of noninsertional Achilles

J.A. Nunley (ed.), *The Achilles Tendon: Treatment and Rehabilitation,*
DOI: 10.1007/978-1-387-79206-4_13, © Springer Science + Business Media, LLC 2009

tendon pain, swelling (diffuse or localized), and impaired performance. Astrom and Rausing[7] recommended use of the term *Achillodynia* as a symptomatic diagnosis, and suggested the terms *peritendonitis* and *tendinosis* be reserved strictly for histopathologic diagnoses.

Noninsertional Achilles tendinopathy can be broadly grouped into either paratendinopathy or intratendinous disease (tendinosis). Achilles paratendinopathy (*peritendonitis/paratendonitis*) is defined as an inflammation of the tissues surrounding the Achilles tendon with histologic specimens showing acute inflammatory features. Clinically, this describes Achilles pain with tenderness to palpation with no intratendinous involvement clinically or on imaging investigations.[5,6]*Tendinosis* is described as the chronic intratendinous degeneration of the tendon with the histologic presence of coalesced collagen fibers, cystic mucoid changes, calcification, and vascular degenerative changes. Despite the label "degenerative," Achilles tendinosis is thought likely to be reversible.[1] While chronic tendinosis exhibits no histologic findings of inflammation, it is unclear whether inflammatory changes are seen in the acute phase. The distinction between the two often cannot be made clinically on history and examination alone.[8,9] These disorders may present as distinct entities or can coexist. To date, there has been no clinical significance to the differentiation of paratendinopathy from intrasubstance tendinosis, as treatment is similar for both groups, and no study to date has compared the outcomes of the two entities.

Classification

Classifications of Achilles tendinopathy, based on location and chronology classification, have been suggested. Noninsertional Achilles pathology may involve the paratenon, the tendon, or both, with simultaneous involvement of the paratenon and the tendon referred to as *pantendinopathy*. Thought to exist on a spectrum, Achilles tendinopathy may also be categorized as acute, subacute, and chronic, based on the duration of symptomatology. Acute tendinopathy is defined as symptoms present for less than 2 weeks, subacute as 2 to 6 weeks, and chronic as greater than 6 weeks.[10] Chronologic classification is purely descriptive and not based on any clinical or pathologic distinction.

Anatomy

The Achilles tendon may be subjected to tensile loads that are ten times body weight during running, jumping, hopping, and skipping.[11–13] Grossly, the Achilles tendon is approximately 15 cm in length and originates from the musculotendinous junction of the gastrocnemius and soleus muscles where it has a flattened shape. As the Achilles tendon travels distally, it becomes increasingly more rounded to a point 4 cm above the insertion before progressively flattening out toward its broad insertion.[14,15]

The Achilles tendon does not have a true tenosynovial sheath, but instead is surrounded by a thin gliding membrane of loose areolar tissue referred to as the *paratenon*. This layer is contiguous with the fascial layer proximally and the calcaneal periosteum distally.[16] Immediately superficial to the posterior paratenon is the crural fascia of the lower leg, with the epitenon being immediately deep to the paratenon. The fluid between the epitenon and paratenon minimizes friction to enable smooth excursion of the Achilles tendon.[17]

Tropocollagen (type I collagen) is arranged longitudinally in line with the length of the tendon. This collagen sequentially forms microfibrils, fibrils, fibers, fascicles, and bundles. The bundles are encased in a loose connective tissue layer called the *endotenon*. The entire tendon is covered by the *epitenon*, an adherent layer continuous with the endotenon. The longitudinal alignment of the collagen fibers imparts tensile strength. There is also a small proportion of fibers that course transversely and in a spiral configuration allowing for resistance to shear and rotation.

Blood vessels, nerves, and lymphatics enter the Achilles tendon from the paratenon via the epitenon and continuous endotenon. The nerves and blood vessels that supply the Achilles tendon travel along the paratenon and enter via the epitenon and eventually the endotenon.[18,19] The majority of the blood supply is from the anterior paratenon.

The area of lowest vascularity is 2 to 6 cm above the calcaneal insertion. This relative watershed area is postulated to be a possible contributing factor to the development of tendinopathy. [20–22] This watershed area has been confirmed by angiographic studies.[18,19] The blood flow diminishes with age and may impair healing with trauma.

Etiology of Achilles Tendinopathy

Extrinsic vs. Intrinsic

Numerous factors have been associated with the development of noninsertional Achilles tendinopathy. The true underlying etiology and natural history of Achilles tendinopathy is currently a topic of investigation. These factors can be broadly classified as intrinsic or extrinsic. While no single etiologic factor can be isolated, it is likely that the process is multifactorial in overuse injuries and predominately extrinsic in acute trauma (Tables 13.1 and 13.2)[23,24].

Table 13.1 Intrinsic factors contributing to Achilles tendinopathy.

General/systemic
    Age
    Gender
    Systemic disease
    Endocrine/metabolic (obesity, estrogen exposure)
Local
    Biomechanical/lower extremity malalignment
    Leg length discrepancy
    Muscular weakness/imbalance

Table 13.2 Extrinsic factors contributing to Achilles tendinopathy.

Medication/drugs
    Corticosteroids
    Anabolic steroids
    Fluoroquinolone antibiotics
Activity factors
Overload/repetitive
    Duration/intensity training
    Rapid progression of training
    Improper footwear
    Fatigue
    Lack of variation in training
    Inadequate warm-up or stretching
Environmental
    Hard training surface
    Cold weather

Intrinsic Factors

Age

The aging process results in a decline in the physiologic proportion of type I collagen as it is gradually replaced by a relatively higher concentration of type III collagen. Type I collagen provides mechanical strength to tension, whereas type III collagen is associated with decreased elasticity and increased weakness to tensile loads. This natural change with age results in histologic tendinopathy predisposing patients to partial tears and subsequent pain.

Chronic Achilles disorders are more prevalent in older athletes than among young athletes.[25] Kvist[26] studied 470 patients with Achilles tendinopathy or insertional complaints, and reported that only 25% were young athletes, and only 10% were younger than 14 years of age.

Gender

The incidence of Achilles tendinopathy is higher in males. It is unclear if this reflects an underlying structural predisposition or a higher predominance of males participating in high-impact activities leading to Achilles tendinopathy.

Systemic Illness

There has been no defined association between Achilles tendinopathy and systemic disease. However, the majority of Achilles injuries are thought to originate from greater than physiologic load or tendon degeneration. Only 2% of injuries are attributed to a systemic condition such as inflammatory arthropathy.[27,28]

Endocrine and Metabolic Factors

Holmes and Lin[29] demonstrated a correlation between obesity, hypertension, steroids, and estrogen exposure with the development of Achilles tendinopathy. Obesity is postulated to cause an insulin-resistant state resulting in diminished endothelial cell nitric oxide levels. Hypertension alters the biomechanical properties of arterial vessels, decreasing compliance and promoting a prothrombotic state. Diabetes mellitus was statistically associated only in men younger than 44 years of age. Holmes and Lin concluded that these systemic factors exerted an influence via the diminution of local microvascularity. These same factors have previously been associated with acute Achilles tendon ruptures and posterior tibial tendon dysfunction.

Biomechanics, Gait, and Lower Extremity Malalignment
Epidemiologic studies demonstrate that nonphysiologic biomechanics, gait, and lower extremity alignment may predispose patients to the development of Achilles tendinopathy. Kvist[3,26] reported a 60% incidence of lower extremity malalignment in his series of chronic Achilles tendon disorders. Marked forefoot varus is found in athletes with Achilles tendon overuse injuries, reflecting the predisposing role played by hyperpronation.[3,26,30,31]

Athletes complaining of Achilles tendinopathy often have limited passive dorsiflexion of the ankle joint with the knee extended and limited passive subtalar joint mobility.[3,26] Kaufman et al.[32] observed that restricted ankle dorsiflexion with the knee in extension and increased hindfoot inversion are associated with Achilles tendinopathy. Despite the association of malalignment and Achilles tendinopathy as noted above, the role that these disorders play in the pathogenesis of tendinopathy remains unclear.[30]

Leg Length Discrepancy
The contribution of limb-length discrepancy to the development of Achilles tendinopathy is controversial. The traditional orthopedic perspective is that discrepancies of less than 20 mm are not clinically important and that a leg length discrepancy of 10 to 20 mm is a common asymptomatic finding in the general population.[30] However, it has been proposed that in elite athletes, a discrepancy of 5 mm can predispose to overuse injuries. At present, the role and the magnitude of the leg length discrepancy in the development of overuse injuries and possible Achilles tendinopathy are unknown.[23]

Muscular Weakness and Imbalance
Muscular weakness and imbalance may contribute to the development of Achilles tendinopathy. By acting as a shock absorber to dissipate forces, optimal muscular strength and flexibility have been shown to protect the musculoskeletal system from impact loading.[23] A lack of strength, endurance, or flexibility will impair this protective mechanism and expose the Achilles tendon to excessive strain and possible tendinopathy. Recent studies have demonstrated symptomatic relief from chronic Achilles tendinopathy in patients rehabilitated with heavy-load eccentric calf training.[33–37] Ninety of 101 patients (89%) had improvement on the visual analogue scale and were back to their preinjury activity levels after the 12-week training regimen.[33,34] The true contribution of muscular pathology to Achilles tendinopathy is debatable, and it is unknown whether the muscular disorder was an underlying cause or a result of the Achilles tendinopathy.

Extrinsic Factors

Overuse/Repetitive Strain
Typically, overuse injuries are seen in repetitive, high-impact activities such as running and jumping. The development of Achilles tendinopathy is highest among those participating in track-and-field events, particularly middle- and

long-distance running. Other activities with a predilection to Achilles disorders are volleyball, soccer, tennis, badminton, and orienteering.[2,3,26,38–40] The annual incidence of Achilles disorders is between 7% and 9%.[2,39] Of these Achilles disorders, tendinopathy is the most common clinical entity, comprising 55% to 65% of cases, followed by insertional problems, comprising 20% to 25% of cases.[1,3,26]

Overuse, repetition, and training errors are regarded as common extrinsic factors in the development of Achilles tendinopathy, reported in 60% to 80% of cases.[3,24,26] Running an excessively long distance, running at too high an intensity, increasing intensity or distance too quickly, excessive uphill or downhill training, and training on sloped surfaces account for the majority of training errors.[3,24,26] Monotonous, asymmetric, and specialized repetitive training in addition to fatigue can also contribute to Achilles disorders.[1] At a mean follow-up of 11 years, Kujala et al.[41] reported 79 of 269 male orienteering runners (29%) complained of an Achilles tendon overuse injury compared to only seven of 188 controls (4%) with an age-adjusted odds ratio of 10.0. In this study, 66% had noninsertional Achilles tendinopathy and 23% had insertional disorders. Paavola et al.[42] demonstrated that those patients presenting with unilateral tendinopathy are at high risk of developing similar symptoms on the contralateral side. In this study, 41% developed similar symptoms on the contralateral side within the 8-year follow-up period.

Environmental

Adverse environmental conditions, including cold weather, hard running surfaces, and slippery/icy surfaces, may also predispose to Achilles disorders.[9,28,30,43] While associated, the majority of these factors have not been directly correlated with Achilles tendon disorders.

Steroids (Local and Systemic)

Traditionally, intratendinous injection of corticosteroids has been associated with tendon degeneration and subsequent rupture; however, there is no strong evidence to support this view.[44] A recent study of five patients demonstrated that corticosteroids injected directly into the tendon of patients with Achilles tendinopathy resulted in satisfactory pain relief without complications.[45] There currently exists no strong evidence to support or condemn intrasubstance injection of corticosteroids. In contrast, the use of anabolic steroids, has been documented to increase the rate of tendinopathy and tendon rupture.[46]

Fluoroquinolone Antibiotics

Despite the relatively large volume of case-based evidence, the pathophysiology of fluoroquinolone-induced tendinopathy and tendon rupture is unclear.[47–50] The effect may be mediated through the fluoroquinolone potentiated interleukin-1 (IL-1) and tumor necrosis factor-α (TNF-α)-stimulated expression of matrix metalloproteinases (MMPs) in human tendon-derived cells.[48,51–53] The degradation of collagen and other extracellular matrix components is initiated by MMPs. The action of MMPs is countered by the inhibitory action of tissue inhibitors of metalloproteinases (TIMPs), which are stimulated by transforming growth factor-β (TGF-β) and IL-6. Any alteration in this delicate balance can lead to collagen and tendon degeneration.[48,51–53]

Pathophysiology of Achilles Tendinopathy

The Achilles tendon responds to supraphysiologic loading with inflammatory changes in the tendon sheath, intratendinous degeneration of the tendon body, or a combination of both. Noninsertional Achilles tendinopathy may be a precursor to Achilles tendon ruptures or may predispose the tendon to rupture.

Peritendinous

Early in the development of paratendinopathy there is an inflammatory phase with edema and subsequent fibrin exudate.[9,28] Both classic fibroblasts and myofibroblast-like cells in the chronically inflamed paratenon tissue are believed to contribute to the clinical symptoms in paratendinopathy. If there is delayed or inadequate healing, the fibrin can organize and form adhesions between the Achilles epitenon and the paratenon, resulting in crepitus, swelling, and pain.[54–56] These changes were noted to impair the gliding function of both the Achilles tendon epitenon-paratenon interval and the paratenon-crural fascial interval.[54–56]

Histologic examination of the peritendinous structures reveals the presence of both fibroblasts and myofibroblasts, comprising up to 20% of the peritendinous cells in chronic paratendinopathy.[54–56] Under mechanical strain, fibroblasts secrete TGF-β that follows a paracrine mechanism to induce tenocyte metaplasia into myofibroblasts, resulting in peritendinous tissue scarring and contraction. This causes a constrictive effect on the local circulation that may leave an area of relative tendon hypovascularity.

Intratendinous

The structure of the tendon is disrupted micro- or macroscopically by repetitive strain. Collagen fibers begin to slide past one another, causing breakage of their cross-linked structure with resultant inflammation, edema, and pain.[23] Any disorganized, haphazard, or incomplete healing can result in chronic tendinopathy.[53,57,58]

On a microcellular level, the degradation of collagen and other extracellular matrix components is initiated by MMPs. The action of MMPs is countered by TIMPs, stimulated by TGF-β and IL-6.[59] The MMPs can be up- or down-regulated at the local and systemic levels.[60,61] Any alteration in this balance can lead to collagen and tendon degeneration.

The production of MMP-1, TIMP-1, and gelatinolytic activities in cell cultures from tendinosis samples and controls has been examined in patellar tendinopathy. Tendinosis tissues showed an increased MMP-1 expression and a decrease in TIMP-1.[62,63] This condition favors collagen degradation and supports a role of imbalance in collagen homeostasis as a causative factor in tendinopathy that may be applicable to Achilles tendinopathy.

The paratenon is richly innervated and vascularized, providing the nerve and blood supply to the Achilles tendon. The nerves accompany the vascular channels within the substance of the tendon itself. Several terminal sensory branches terminate in the tendon. It is postulated that both the neovascularization and the multiple sensory nerve ending may be responsible for the pain experienced in Achilles tendinopathy.[45,64–66]

Diagnosis

History

A focused but detailed history should identify the onset, frequency, and duration of symptoms. Any contributing factors such as changes in activity level, shoe wear, potential training errors, and previous treatment modalities should be elicited. It is imperative to recognize the patient's expectations regarding his desired level of activity.

Classically, noninsertional Achilles tendinopathy presents as a pain with activation occurring 2 to 6 cm proximal to the Achilles insertion in essentially the same location as Achilles tendon ruptures. While noninsertional Achilles tendinopathy is typically experienced only during physically demanding sporting activities, the pain can progress to eventually affect daily activities. There is a correlation between severity of tendinopathy and the degree of morning stiffness.[67] Runners complain of pain at the beginning and end of training, but often with a characteristic pain-free period in the middle of the activity.[68]

In addition, partial or complete ruptures of the Achilles tendon should always be suspected. Typically, the acuity of onset distinguishes ruptures from noninsertional tendinopathy, with the former presenting with a sudden onset and the latter with gradual onset.

Physical Examination

Although disorders of the Achilles are described as distinct entities, many disorders exhibit a variety of symptoms and may reflect the presence of more than one disorder simultaneously (Table 13.3).

However, the differentiation between insertional and noninsertional tendinopathy can generally be readily made. Examination should start with proper exposure of bilateral lower extremities. In a standing position, assessment of lower limb alignment, leg length discrepancy, and gait is noted. Approximately 60% of patients with chronic Achilles tendinopathy have lower extremity malalignment.[3,26] The posterior leg is then examined for symmetry, atrophy, nodular thickening, and previous incisions. After inspection, the leg is palpated for the point of maximum tenderness and any swelling or irregularity (Fig. 13.1).

Table 13.3 Physical exam findings in Achilles tendon disorders.

Pain/tenderness/swelling location insertional/noninsertional focal vs. diffuse swelling
Acuity of onset (gradual/sudden)
Morning stiffness/pain
Palpable gap
Crepitus
Thompson test
Painful arc sign
Royal London hospital test

Fig. 13.1. Noninsertional Achilles tendinopathy typically presents as a tender, fusiform thickening of the Achilles tendon 4 to 7 cm proximal to the tendon's insertion on the calcaneus

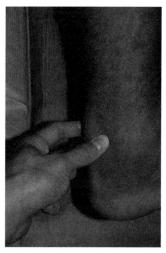

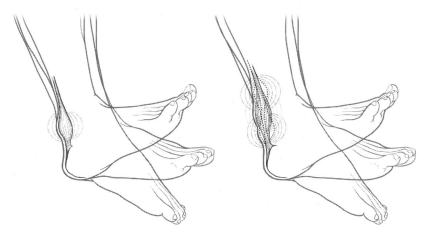

Fig. 13.2. The painful arc sign is a clinical exam finding that may distinguish tendinopathy from paratendinopathy. With ankle range of motion, tenderness remains in a fixed location with paratendinopathy, but demonstrates migration that corresponds to the motion of the ankle. (Adapted from Williams,[16] with permission from Wolters Kluwer Health.)

The ankle and subtalar joint are then placed through a range of motion, taking note of any crepitus or restricted range of motion. Patients with Achilles tendinopathy often have limited passive dorsiflexion of the ankle joint, with the knee extended limitation of passive subtalar joint mobility.[3,26] The peritendinous fibrous exudates, adhesions, and thickening of the paratenon found in paratendinopathy may present with crepitus during fast up-and-down motion. Tendon adhesions and thickening of the paratenon are not observed in tendinosis.[53,68] These findings are typically noted with isolated tendinopathy, but may be observed in pantendinopathy (Fig. 13.2).

The painful-arc sign is a physical finding in patients with tendinopathy whereby a tender area of intratendinous swelling moves relative to the malleoli with the tendon during ankle dorsiflexion and plantarflexion, indicating the presence of intrasubstance tendon pathology. In contrast, paratendinopathy patients exhibit a painful thickening that remains fixed in position relative to the malleoli throughout ankle range of motion.[16,69]

Lastly, the Royal London Hospital test is described as the significant decrease or disappearance of tenderness when the tendon is placed under tension. This test is considered specific for intrasubstance tendinopathy.[70]

For completeness, the exam should include careful palpation of the tendon, not only for nodules or fusiform swelling, but also for partial or complete defects. Rarely, an Achilles tendon rupture may present with a history consistent with tendinopathy, particularly with the intact function of the other flexors of the ankle. A Thompson test should be routinely performed. While chronic Achilles tendinopathy may lead to tendon attenuation, it generally does not present with a positive Thompson test. A positive test suggests Achilles rupture, perhaps with associated Achilles degeneration.

Imaging Modalities

Imaging is used to delineate the extent and severity of intratendinous degeneration in addition to differentiating between intrasubstance tendinopathy and paratendinopathy.

X-Rays

Conventional plain radiography is readily accessible, but is limited in imaging the soft tissue structures of the Achilles tendon. The anterior border of the Achilles tendon is well delineated because of the adjacent pre-Achilles fat pad, which is relatively radiolucent. Occasionally, in cases of Achilles tendinopathy or rupture, this well-defined anterior border of the Achilles tendon is blurred on lateral radiographs.[71] Occasionally, Achilles pathology develops into calcific tendinosis. These calcifications are readily visible on plain x-ray.

Ultrasound

Advances in ultrasound, including higher frequency transducers, better image resolution, and improved field of view, have expanded the role of ultrasound in the diagnosis and management of Achilles tendon disorders. Current ultrasonographic devices afford considerable clarity and accuracy in the diagnosis of soft tissue disorders, rivaling data obtained in older low-tesla magnetic resonance imaging (MRI) units.

Ultrasound is a reliable, inexpensive, and readily accessible modality for evaluating the Achilles tendon. It has the unique ability to perform dynamic real-time visualization of the tendon, permitting assessment of the gliding motion of the Achilles tendon. The experience and skill of the ultrasonographer often dictates the value and yield of the diagnostic test. Thus, if treating surgeons wish to utilize this technology in their practice, specialized training typically is needed. Alternatively, real-time data may be obtained and stored by the radiologist for later review by the treating surgeon.

On transverse imaging, the physiologically normal Achilles tendon has a flat to concave anterior surface and measures 4 to 6 mm in anterior to posterior dimension.[72–75] The tendon dimensions increase to 7 to 16 mm in patients with intrasubstance tendinopathy.[72] Athletes with intrasubstance tendinopathy demonstrate an Achilles tendon that is on average 78% thicker than the contralateral side.[76]

In acute paratendinopathy, fluid is often present surrounding the Achilles tendon. In chronic paratendinopathy, adhesions can be seen as a thickening of the hypoechogenic paratenon with poorly defined borders and a normal tendon. However, there is the risk of a false negative if adhesions are not found or not present.[77,78]

In general, ultrasound findings correlate well with histopathologic findings.[8,79,80] The ultrasound finding of a heterogeneous tendon may be predictive of outcome in patients with painful Achilles tendinopathy.[81,82] Furthermore, the appearance of a normal Achilles tendon on ultrasound is associated with a better clinical outcome in patients with a clinical diagnosis of Achilles tendinopathy compared to those with an abnormal ultrasound appearance.[83]

Lastly, the information gleaned from ultrasound may be enhanced with the addition of color Doppler imaging. Color Doppler imaging is suggestive of neovascularization in Achilles tendinopathy. While neovascularization may be construed to be an indication of tendon healing, it is probably more consistent with symptomatic tendinopathy, with a negative effect on patient outcome, particularly with nonoperative management.[82] Neovascularization typically is accompanied by ingrowth of sensory nerve fibers into the area of tendinopathy.

Magnetic Resonance Imaging

Magnetic resonance imaging has been the imaging modality of choice because of its ability to provide clear and accurate detailed images in multiple planes. Limitations of MRI are cost, lack of the immediate real-time dynamic images afforded by ultrasonography, and potential false-positive interpretation of suspected findings.

The physiologic anteroposterior (AP) dimension of the Achilles tendon on MRI is 6 mm.[75] The anterior aspect of the tendon is flat to concave. The normal Achilles tendon appears black on all MRI sequences because of its low water content and the compact alignment of collagen fibers.

In Achilles intrasubstance tendinopathy, the tendon often takes a fusiform shape with thickening and loss of the anterior concavity (Fig. 13.3). Areas

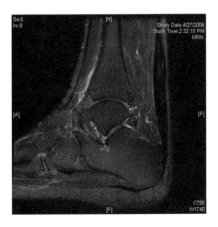 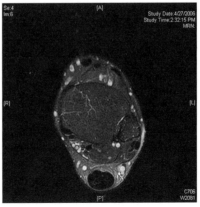

A   B

Fig. 13.3. (A) T2–weighted sagittal image demonstrates signal change within the Achilles tendon proximal to the tendon's insertion on the calcaneus and defines the extent of tendinopathy. (B) T2–weighted axial image demonstrates the extent of signal change within the tendon at the site of tendinopathy

of increased intrasubstance signal can be seen on both T1- and T2-weighted images.[84–86] The sensitivity and specificity of MRI in detecting abnormalities in painful Achilles tendinopathy is 94% and 81%, respectively.[84,85]

However, as a result of its enhanced sensitivity, the presence of altered signals may lead to the diagnosis and treatment of asymptomatic disorders. Magnetic resonance imaging findings seen in patients with painful tendinopathy are also seen in patients who are asymptomatic.[87,88] The significance of post-operative signal abnormalities remains undefined.[84,87,88]

Treatment

A poor understanding of the natural history of noninsertional tendinopathy contributes to a lack of full understanding of the role of intervention. The multitude of conservative and surgical treatment strategies advocated for noninsertional tendinopathy implies a lack of a single definitive treatment approach. Treatment is largely supported only by retrospective data and empirically derived algorithms rather than evidence-based outcome studies. This discussion focuses on nonoperative management of paratendinopathy and intrasubstance tendinopathy; Chapter 16 discusses the surgical treatment of noninsertional Achilles tendinopathy.

Conservative Treatment

Treatment is targeted at correcting the intrinsic and extrinsic contributing factors to relieve or modify symptoms. The majority of patients with a painful noninsertional tendinopathy can be successfully treated without surgical intervention.

The longest longitudinal data were reported by Paavola et al.,[42] whose 83 patients with acute or subacute Achilles tendinopathy were treated conservatively for an average of 8 years. Seventy patients (84%) had full recovery of their activity level, and 78 patients (94%) were asymptomatic or had only mild pain with strenuous exercise at final follow-up. The analysis included a questionnaire, clinical examination, performance tests, muscle strength measurement, and ultrasonographic examination. In addition, the same authors demonstrated that 41% of patients with Achilles tendinopathy developed overuse symptoms of the contralateral Achilles tendon during the 8-year follow-up period. Despite the apparent success with nonoperative management, 24 of the 83 patients (29%) needed surgery during the follow-up period, because of an inability of conservative measures to relieve symptoms adequately.[42] Moreover, other studies have suggested a higher failure rate of 35% to 50% with nonsurgical management.[6,89]

Physical Therapy

Physical therapy techniques focusing on concentric strengthening, eccentric strengthening, stretching, and numerous other modalities have been reported in the treatment of noninsertional Achilles tendinopathy. In our experience, an aggressive stretching protocol may aggravate the symptoms. We typically recommend a supervised physical therapy protocol with modalities that eventually are transferred to a patient-maintained home program.

Modalities

Modalities including cold and heat therapy,[28] massage, ultrasound, electrical stimulation,[90] and laser therapy[91] have been used, but with little supportive evidence to substantiate their benefit and role.

Iontophoresis is a noninvasive method of introducing high concentrations of a drug into a joint or small body part via electrical current. The application of a charge to the skin alters the skin's permeability increasing migration of the drug to depths of 1 to 2 cm.[92] The most commonly used drugs are steroids and antiinflammatories. This has been demonstrated to have beneficial effects in multiple musculoskeletal disorders,[90,93,94] but its specific role and benefits in the treatment of Achilles tendinopathy is limited.[95,96]

Eccentric Strengthening

Heavy load eccentric calf muscle strengthening has demonstrated, in well-designed studies, excellent results in the treatment of noninsertional Achilles tendinopathy.[33,97–99] Eccentric strengthening is superior to concentric strengthening in alleviating pain in chronic Achilles tendinopathy, with 81% to 89% of patients studied reporting resolution of symptoms.[33,99] The mechanism allowing for resolution of symptoms is an increase in tensile strength of the tendon or by lengthening of the muscle tendon unit by stretch, resulting in less strain with ankle motion.

The initial prospective study of eccentric strengthening for noninsertional Achilles tendinopathy had 15 recreational athletes with calf pain and swelling localized 2 to 6 cm from the insertion; noninsertional tendinopathy was confirmed by ultrasound. An eccentric stretching program, consisting of 15 eccentric heel drops twice a day, 7 days a week, for 12 weeks, was used. The exercise was meant to be painful. If no pain was experienced, the load was increased until pain was experienced. After 12 weeks, all 15 patients were satisfied and had returned to their preinjury levels of activity.[33]

A subsequent study found satisfactory results in 90 of 101 tendons with chronic noninsertional Achilles tendinopathy.[34] Similar benefit has not been shown for this technique in patients with insertional Achilles tendinopathy. Follow-up ultrasonographic examination of these patients with eccentric strengthening demonstrated that the Achilles tendon thickness decreased, and the tendon appearance was more physiologic than before treatment.[35]

Correction of Malalignment/Leg Length Discrepancy

Kvist[3,26] reported a 60% incidence of lower extremity malalignment in his series of chronic Achilles tendon disorders. Marked forefoot varus is found in athletes with Achilles tendon overuse injuries, reflecting the predisposing role hyperpronation plays.[3,26,30,31] Orthotics and shoe wear modifications have been used without any strong data to support their role in altering the natural history of Achilles tendinopathy. While some authors propose that a leg-length discrepancy of 5 mm can predispose to overuse injuries in elite athletes, at present, the role and magnitude of the leg length discrepancy in the development of overuse injuries and possible Achilles tendinopathy is unknown.[23]

Heel Lifts

Heel lifts have been advocated as a means to remove excessive tension from the Achilles tendon and thereby minimize irritation and pain from Achilles tendinopathy.[100] A heel lift of 1 inch can decrease plantarflexion muscle torque by nearly 50%.[101]

Activity Modification and Training Factors

Training errors,[102–104], muscle weakness,[28,105] decreased flexibility,[11,28] and poor equipment[33,102] have been implicated as important etiologic factors requiring treatment to alleviate painful Achilles tendinopathy. While we agree that the initial treatment strategy of Achilles tendinopathy should include the identification and correction of these errors, the evidence to support these strategies is based only on retrospective studies, expert opinion, and anecdotal experience.

Nonsteroidal Antiinflammatory Drugs

While nonsteroidal antiinflammatory drugs (NSAIDs) may provide symptomatic relief in the acute phase of tendon pathology, there is little evidence that they contribute to the resolution of tendinopathy. Recent evidence has failed to demonstrate the presence of any inflammatory markers in chronic Achilles tendinopathy, questioning the role of NSAIDs in management. Histologic biopsy of patients with chronic midportion Achilles tendinopathy failed to demonstrate any inflammatory cell infiltration.[97] Astrom and Westlin[106] reported the results of a double-blinded, placebo-controlled trial to examine the effects of NSAIDs on 70 consecutive adult, nonrheumatic patients with a painful Achilles tendinopathy. Patients were randomized to receive either piroxicam or placebo. Both groups received adjunct treatment with a period of rest combined with stretching and strengthening exercises. No differences were seen between the groups at any time during the study. Furthermore, recent studies demonstrate that NSAIDs may impair tendon healing via stimulation of increased intratendinous leukotriene B4 levels.[107] NSAIDs may still have a role in the acute phase and are still often advocated. They offer symptomatic relief, but do not result in definitive resolution of the underlying tendinopathy.

Corticosteroids

Concerns regarding the association of peritendinous injection and tendon rupture are based on retrospective data and case reports only. While the majority of sources recommend avoiding intratendinous injection because of the risk of subsequent further degeneration and rupture,[45,108,109] corticosteroid injecions are commonly used in the treatment of chronic tendon disorders.[110–112] Fluoroscopically guided low-volume peritendinous corticosteroid injection showed no major complication or rupture.[94] A meta-analysis and retrospective study of cortisone peritendinous injection for Achilles tendinopathy concluded that there were insufficient data to determine the risk of rupture.[113] Nonetheless, partial ruptures have been reported after steroid injection.[114,115]

Despite widespread and liberal use, the physiologic basis of their effect and the systematic evidence for their benefits are largely lacking. A distinction

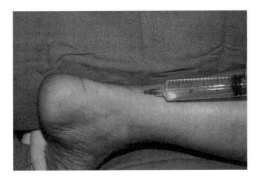

Fig.13.4. Brisement—or injection of saline with or without anesthetic—between the paratenon and Achilles tendon may release symptomatic adhesions that create a condition analogous to stenosing flexor tenosynovitis. Brisement may be combined with ultrasound to better locate the area of greatest disease and to better direct the injection between the paratenon and Achilles tendon

between peritendinous and intratendinous injection should be made. For peritendinous injection, the corticosteroid acts as a potent suppressor of inflammation and may inhibit adhesion and scar tissue formation. The results of peritendinous injection remain inconclusive, with one series reporting a 40% improvement[94] and another study demonstrating no improvement compared to placebo.[112] Focused, often ultrasound-guided, intrasubstance injection has not been widely studied; only smaller retrospective studies have assessed intratendinous injection.[45] There is insufficient evidence to support or refute the role of focused intratendinous injection (Fig. 13.4) .

Alternative Injections

Low-dose heparin, glycosaminoglycans, and aprotinin have been advocated for both intrasubstance tendinosis and paratendinopathy. There are insufficient data to support their use.[64,116] Hyaluronan is a high-molecular-weight polysaccharide normally found in synovial fluid around tendon sheaths. The benefit of injection is believed to be secondary to the decrease in adhesion formation. While benefit has been shown in rabbit flexor tendons, no such benefit has been demonstrated in a rat Achilles tendon model.[117,118] This may be due to a lack of a true synovial sheath around the Achilles tendon as mentioned earlier.

Sclerosing Agents

One theory of the pathogenesis of painful noninsertional Achilles tendinopathy implicates neovascularization associated with pain generation. This presence has been documented on both ultrasound and color Doppler studies.[64,66] Ablation of these neovessels has been postulated to alleviate the pain associated with Achilles tendinopathy.[64,66] Injection of a sclerosing agent (polidocanol) in the area of neovascularization provided pain relief in eight of 10 patients at 6 months and at 2 years.[64] Although sclerosing agents are injected to target neovascularization, elimination of accompanying sensory nerve endings may provide the greatest symptomatic relief, thus perhaps explaining this seemingly counterintuitive approach. It is uncertain if this therapy promotes healing or is limited to relief of symptoms.

Vasodilation Techniques

Nitric oxide, reported to contribute to fracture and wound healing by potentially increasing microcirculation and stimulating fibroblast collagen synthesis, has also been applied to the management of tendinopathy.[119–121] Glyceryl trinitrate is a commonly used drug that undergoes denitration in the body to become an active metabolite (nitric oxide).

A prospective randomized, double-blind, placebo-controlled trial of 65 patients (84 Achilles tendons) compared continuous application of topical glyceryl trinitrate with rehabilitation alone for the management of noninsertional Achilles tendinopathy. The glyceryl trinitrate group experienced reduced pain and improved outcomes, with 78% of tendons being asymptomatic with activities of daily living at 6 months compared to 49% in the placebo group. At 3 years, this same group receiving the glyceryl nitrate continued to demonstrate less Achilles tendon pain compared to placebo.[122,123] Headaches can be a potential side effect of the glyceryl nitrate treatment. In one study, 17 of 32 patients (53%) experienced headaches, with the majority having symptoms within the first 2 weeks of treatment.[122,123] Only one patient of the 17 had to discontinue use of the glyceryl nitrate due to persistent headaches.[122,123]

Pulsed Electromagnetic Fields

Pulsed electromagnetic fields (PEMFs) may enhance calcium binding in the growth factor cascades responsible for tissue healing. In the rat Achilles tendon model, a PEMF results in an increase of the Achilles tendon's tensile strength.[124] Pulsed magnetic fields (17 Hz) have been applied to rat Achilles tendinopathy models, resulting in an improved alignment of collagen fibers.[125] Low-intensity electrical pulsed galvanic current in tenotomized rat tendons demonstrated increased force to breakage in the anode-stimulated group compared to the control group.[126]

Extracorporeal Shock Wave

Extracorporeal shock wave (ECSW) has been studied in various tendon disorders of the musculoskeletal system including rotator cuff pathology and patellar tendinopathy.[127–129] It has also been studied in both insertional and noninsertional Achilles tendinopathy.[130–132] Some evidence in the rat model resulted in promotion of tendon healing believed to be secondary to increased levels of TGF-β1 in the early stage and persistent elevation of insulin-like growth factor I (IGF-I).[133]

Furia[132] compared the effects of a single-dose high-energy shock wave in 34 patients with noninsertional Achilles tendinopathy to a control group of 34 patients. At 12 months, there was a statistically significant difference in successful outcomes, favoring the high-energy shock wave group. Extracorporeal shock wave can, however, result in dose-dependent tendon damage, including fibrinoid necrosis, fibrosis, and inflammation shown in rabbit models. Extracorporeal shock wave should be used with caution.[134]

Presently, there is great interest in the role of ECSW in the treatment of Achilles tendinopathy. There is insufficient evidence to draw any conclusions regarding the role of ECSW specifically in noninsertional Achilles tendinopathy.

Conclusion

Nonoperative management remains the first-line treatment for noninsertional Achilles tendinopathy. We do not yet have a full understanding of the natural history and pathogenesis of Achilles paratendinopathy and tendinopathy, and most nonoperative treatment is largely unsubstantiated and based on poor evidence. Prospective, randomized trials will determine if our current nonsurgical treatment is justified. Future directions include cytokines, growth factors, gene therapy, tissue engineering, and stem cell research.

References

1. Jarvinen TA, Kannus P, Maffulli N, Khan KM. Achilles tendon disorders: etiology and epidemiology. Foot Ankle Clin 2005;10(2):255–66.
2. Johansson C. Injuries in elite orienteers. Am J Sports Med 1986;14(5):410–5.
3. Kvist M. Achilles tendon injuries in athletes. Sports Med 1994;18(3):173–201.
4. Clain MR, Baxter DE. Achilles tendinitis. Foot Ankle 1992;13(8):482–7.
5. Khan KM, Cook JL, Kannus P, Maffulli N, Bonar SF. Time to abandon the "tendinitis" myth. BMJ 2002;324(7338):626–7.
6. Maffulli N, Khan KM, Puddu G. Overuse tendon conditions: time to change a confusing terminology. Arthroscopy 1998;14(8):840–3.
7. Astrom M, Rausing A. Chronic Achilles tendinopathy. A survey of surgical and histopathologic findings. Clin Orthop Rel Res 1995(316):151–64.
8. Kader D, Saxena A, Movin T, Maffulli N. Achilles tendinopathy: some aspects of basic science and clinical management. Br J Sports Med 2002;36(4):239–49.
9. Paavola M, Kannus P, Jarvinen TA, Khan K, Jozsa L, Jarvinen M. Achilles tendinopathy. J Bone Joint Surg [Am] 2002;84–A(11):2062–76.
10. el Hawary R, Stanish WD, Curwin SL. Rehabilitation of tendon injuries in sport. Sports Med 1997;24(5):347–58.
11. Clement DB, Taunton JE, Smart GW. Achilles tendinitis and peritendinitis: etiology and treatment. Am J Sports Med 1984;12(3):179–84.
12. Smart GW, Taunton JE, Clement DB. Achilles tendon disorders in runners—a review. Med Sci Sports Exerc 1980;12(4):231–43.
13. Soma CA, Mandelbaum BR. Achilles tendon disorders. Clin Sports Med 1994;13(4):811–23.
14. O'Brien M. The anatomy of the Achilles tendon. Foot Ankle Clin 2005;10(2):225–38.
15. O'Brien M. Functional anatomy and physiology of tendons. Clin Sports Med 1992;11(3):505–20.
16. Williams JG. Achilles tendon lesions in sport. Sports Med 1986;3(2):114–35.
17. Romanelli DA AL, Mandelbaum BR. Achilles rupture in the athlete; current science and treatment. Sports Med Arthroscopy Rev 2000(8):377–86.
18. Zantop T, Tillmann B, Petersen W. Quantitative assessment of blood vessels of the human Achilles tendon: an immunohistochemical cadaver study. Arch Orthop Trauma Surg 2003;123(9):501–4.
19. Lagergren C, Lindholm A. Vascular distribution in the Achilles tendon; an angiographic and microangiographic study. Acta Chir Scand 1959;116(5–6):491–5.
20. Ahmed IM, Lagopoulos M, McConnell P, Soames RW, Sefton GK. Blood supply of the Achilles tendon. J Orthop Res 1998;16(5):591–6.

21. Carr AJ, Norris SH. The blood supply of the calcaneal tendon. J Bone Joint Surg [Br] 1989;71(1):100–1.
22. Kvist M, Jozsa L, Jarvinen M. Vascular changes in the ruptured Achilles tendon and paratenon. Int Orthop 1992;16(4):377–82.
23. Kannus P. Etiology and pathophysiology of chronic tendon disorders in sports. Scand J Med Sci Sports 1997;7(2):78–85.
24. Jarvinen TA, Kannus P, Paavola M, Jarvinen TL, Jozsa L, Jarvinen M. Achilles tendon injuries. Curr Opin Rheumatol 2001;13(2):150–5.
25. Kannus P, Niittymaki S, Jarvinen M, Lehto M. Sports injuries in elderly athletes: a three-year prospective, controlled study. Age Ageing 1989;18(4):263–70.
26. Kvist M. Achilles tendon injuries in athletes. Ann Chir Gynaecol 1991;80(2):188–201.
27. Kannus P, Jozsa L. Histopathological changes preceding spontaneous rupture of a tendon. J Bone Joint Surg [Am] 1991;73:1507–25.
28. Jozsa L, Kannus P. Human Tendons: Anatomy, Physiology, and Pathology. Champaign, IL, Human Kineties. 1997.
29. Holmes GB, Lin J. Etiologic factors associated with symptomatic Achilles tendinopathy. Foot Ankle Int 2006;27(11):952–9.
30. Nigg BM, Wakeling JM. Impact forces and muscle tuning: a new paradigm. Exerc Sport Sci Rev 2001;29(1):37–41.
31. McCrory JL, Martin DF, Lowery RB, et al. Etiologic factors associated with Achilles tendinitis in runners. Med Sci Sports Exerc 1999;31(10):1374–81.
32. Kaufman KR, Brodine SK, Shaffer RA, Johnson CW, Cullison TR. The effect of foot structure and range of motion on musculoskeletal overuse injuries. Am J Sports Med 1999;27(5):585–93.
33. Alfredson H, Pietila T, Jonsson P, Lorentzon R. Heavy-load eccentric calf muscle training for the treatment of chronic Achilles tendinosis. Am J Sports Med 1998;26(3):360–6.
34. Fahlstrom M, Jonsson P, Lorentzon R, Alfredson H. Chronic Achilles tendon pain treated with eccentric calf-muscle training. Knee Surg Sports Traumatol Arthrosc 2003;11(5):327–33.
35. Ohberg L, Lorentzon R, Alfredson H. Eccentric training in patients with chronic Achilles tendinosis: normalised tendon structure and decreased thickness at follow up. Br J Sports Med 2004;38(1):8–11.
36. Roos EM, Engstrom M, Lagerquist A, Soderberg B. Clinical improvement after 6 weeks of eccentric exercise in patients with mid-portion Achilles tendinopathy— a randomized trial with 1–year follow-up. Scand J Med Sci Sports 2004;14(5):286–95.
37. Shalabi A, Kristoffersen-Wilberg M, Svensson L, Aspelin P, Movin T. Eccentric training of the gastrocnemius-soleus complex in chronic Achilles tendinopathy results in decreased tendon volume and intratendinous signal as evaluated by MRI. Am J Sports Med 2004;32(5):1286–96.
38. Fahlstrom M, Lorentzon R, Alfredson H. Painful conditions in the Achilles tendon region in elite badminton players. Am J Sports Med 2002;30(1):51–4.
39. Leppilahti J, Orava S, Karpakka J, Takala T. Overuse injuries of the Achilles tendon. Ann Chir Gynaecol 1991;80(2):202–7.
40. Lysholm J, Wiklander J. Injuries in runners. Am J Sports Med 1987;15(2):168–71.
41. Kujala UM, Sarna S, Kaprio J. Cumulative incidence of achilles tendon rupture and tendinopathy in male former elite athletes. Clin J Sport Med 2005;15(3):133–5.
42. Paavola M, Kannus P, Paakkala T, Pasanen M, Jarvinen M. Long-term prognosis of patients with Achilles tendinopathy. An observational 8–year follow-up study. Am J Sports Med 2000;28(5):634–42.
43. Milgrom C, Finestone A, Zin D, Mandel D, Novack V. Cold weather training: a risk factor for Achilles paratendinitis among recruits. Foot Ankle Int 2003;24(5):398–401.

44. Paavola M, Kannus P, Jarvinen TA, Jarvinen TL, Jozsa L, Jarvinen M. Treatment of tendon disorders. Is there a role for corticosteroid injection? Foot Ankle Clin 2002;7(3):501–13.
45. Konig MJ T-PS, Qvistgaard E. Preliminary results of colour Doppler guided intratendinous glucocorticoid injection for Achilles tendinosis in 5 patients. Scand J Med Sci Sports 2004;14(2):100–6.
46. Laseter JT, Russell JA. Anabolic steroid-induced tendon pathology: a review of the literature. Med Sci Sports Exerc 1991;23(1):1–3.
47. Ribard P, Audisio F, Kahn MF, et al. Seven Achilles tendinitis including 3 complicated by rupture during fluoroquinolone therapy. J Rheumatol 1992;19(9):1479–81.
48. Pierfitte C, Royer RJ. Tendon disorders with fluoroquinolones. Therapie 1996;51(4):419–20.
49. Khaliq Y, Zhanel GG. Fluoroquinolone-associated tendinopathy: a critical review of the literature. Clin Infect Dis 2003;36(11):1404–10.
50. Kowatari K, Nakashima K, Ono A, Yoshihara M, Amano M, Toh S. Levofloxacin-induced bilateral Achilles tendon rupture: a case report and review of the literature. J Orthop Sci 2004;9(2):186–90.
51. Corps AN, Curry VA, Harrall RL, Dutt D, Hazleman BL, Riley GP. Ciprofloxacin reduces the stimulation of prostaglandin E(2) output by interleukin-1beta in human tendon-derived cells. Rheumatology (Oxford) 2003;42(11):1306–10.
52. Corps AN, Harrall RL, Curry VA, Fenwick SA, Hazleman BL, Riley GP. Ciprofloxacin enhances the stimulation of matrix metalloproteinase 3 expression by interleukin-1beta in human tendon-derived cells. A potential mechanism of fluoroquinolone-induced tendinopathy. Arthritis Rheum 2002;46(11):3034–40.
53. Magra M, Maffulli N. Molecular events in tendinopathy: a role for metalloproteases. Foot Ankle Clin 2005;10(2):267–77.
54. Kvist M, Jozsa L, Jarvinen M, Kvist H. Fine structural alterations in chronic Achilles paratenonitis in athletes. Pathol Res Pract 1985;180(4):416–23.
55. Kvist M, Jozsa L, Jarvinen MJ, Kvist H. Chronic Achilles paratenonitis in athletes: a histological and histochemical study. Pathology 1987;19(1):1–11.
56. Kvist MH, Lehto MU, Jozsa L, Jarvinen M, Kvist HT. Chronic Achilles paratenonitis. An immunohistologic study of fibronectin and fibrinogen. Am J Sports Med 1988;16(6):616–23.
57. Rolf C, Movin T. Etiology, histopathology, and outcome of surgery in achillodynia. Foot Ankle Int 1997;18(9):565–9.
58. Tallon C, Maffulli N, Ewen SW. Ruptured Achilles tendons are significantly more degenerated than tendinopathic tendons. Med Sci Sports Exerc 2001;33(12):1983–90.
59. Gomez DE, Alonso DF, Yoshiji H, Thorgeirsson UP. Tissue inhibitors of metalloproteinases: structure, regulation and biological functions. Eur J Cell Biol 1997;74(2):111–22.
60. Alfredson H, Lorentzon M, Backman S, Backman A, Lerner UH. cDNA-arrays and real-time quantitative PCR techniques in the investigation of chronic Achilles tendinosis. J Orthop Res 2003;21(6):970–5.
61. Ireland D, Harrall R, Curry V, et al. Multiple changes in gene expression in chronic human Achilles tendinopathy. Matrix Biol 2001;20(3):159–69.
62. Cilli F, Khan M, Fu F, Wang JH. Prostaglandin E2 affects proliferation and collagen synthesis by human patellar tendon fibroblasts. Clin J Sport Med 2004;14(4):232–6.
63. Wang JH, Iosifidis MI, Fu FH. Biomechanical basis for tendinopathy. Clin Orthop Rel Res 2006;443:320–32.
64. Ohberg L, Alfredson H. Ultrasound guided sclerosis of neovessels in painful chronic Achilles tendinosis: pilot study of a new treatment. Br J Sports Med 2002;36(3):173–5; discussion 6–7.

65. Ohberg L, Alfredson H. Effects on neovascularisation behind the good results with eccentric training in chronic mid-portion Achilles tendinosis? Knee Surg Sports Traumatol Arthrosc 2004;12(5):465–70.

66. Ohberg L, Lorentzon R, Alfredson H. Neovascularisation in Achilles tendons with painful tendinosis but not in normal tendons: an ultrasonographic investigation. Knee Surg Sports Traumatol Arthrosc 2001;9(4):233–8.

67. Binfield PM, Maffulli N. Surgical management of common tendinopathies of the lower limb. Sports Exerc Injury 1997;3:116–22.

68. Vora AM, Myerson MS, Oliva F, Maffulli N. Tendinopathy of the main body of the Achilles tendon. Foot Ankle Clin 2005;10(2):293–308.

69. Williams JG. Achilles tendon lesions in sport. Sports Med 1993;16(3):216–20.

70. Maffulli N, Kenward MG, Testa V, Capasso G, Regine R, King JB. Clinical diagnosis of Achilles tendinopathy with tendinosis. Clin J Sport Med 2003;13(1):11–5.

71. Fischer. Low Kilovolt Radiography. Philadelphia: WB Saunders, 1981.

72. Fornage BD. Achilles tendon: US examination. Radiology 1986;159(3): 759–64.

73. Kainberger FM, Engel A, Barton P, Huebsch P, Neuhold A, Salomonowitz E. Injury of the Achilles tendon: diagnosis with sonography. AJR Am J Roentgenol 1990;155(5):1031–6.

74. Civeira F, Castillo JJ, Calvo C, et al. [Achilles tendon size by high resolution sonography in healthy population. Relationship with lipid levels]. Med Clin (Barc) 1998;111(2):41–4.

75. Koivunen-Niemela T, Parkkola K. Anatomy of the Achilles tendon (tendo calcaneus) with respect to tendon thickness measurements. Surg Radiol Anat 1995;17(3):263–8.

76. Maffulli N, Regine R, Angelillo M, Capasso G, Filice S. Ultrasound diagnosis of Achilles tendon pathology in runners. Br J Sports Med 1987;21(4):158–62.

77. Laine HR, Harjula AL, Peltokallio P. Ultrasonography as a differential diagnostic aid in achillodynia. J Ultrasound Med 1987;6(7):351–62.

78. Paavola M, Paakkala T, Kannus P, Jarvinen M. Ultrasonography in the differential diagnosis of Achilles tendon injuries and related disorders. A comparison between pre-operative ultrasonography and surgical findings. Acta Radiol 1998;39(6): 612–9.

79. Movin T, Gad A, Guntner P, Foldhazy Z, Rolf C. Pathology of the Achilles tendon in association with ciprofloxacin treatment. Foot Ankle Int 1997;18(5):297–9.

80. Movin T, Guntner P, Gad A, Rolf C. Ultrasonography-guided percutaneous core biopsy in Achilles tendon disorder. Scand J Med Sci Sports 1997;7(4):244–8.

81. Archambault JM, Wiley JP, Bray RC, Verhoef M, Wiseman DA, Elliott PD. Can sonography predict the outcome in patients with achillodynia? J Clin Ultrasound 1998;26(7):335–9.

82. Zanetti M, Metzdorf A, Kundert HP, et al. Achilles tendons: clinical relevance of neovascularization diagnosed with power Doppler US. Radiology 2003;227(2) 556–60.

83. Nehrer S, Breitenseher M, Brodner W, et al. Clinical and sonographic evaluation of the risk of rupture in the Achilles tendon. Arch Orthop Trauma Surg 1997;116(1–2):14–8.

84. Karjalainen PT, Ahovuo J, Pihlajamaki HK, Soila K, Aronen HJ. Postoperative MR imaging and ultrasonography of surgically repaired Achilles tendon ruptures. Acta Radiol 1996;37(5):639–46.

85. Karjalainen PT, Aronen HJ, Pihlajamaki HK, Soila K, Paavonen T, Bostman OM. Magnetic resonance imaging during healing of surgically repaired Achilles tendon ruptures. Am J Sports Med 1997;25(2):164–71.

86. Schweitzer ME, Karasick D. MR imaging of disorders of the Achilles tendon. AJR Am J Roentgenol 2000;175(3):613–25.

87. Haims AH, Schweitzer ME, Patel RS, Hecht P, Wapner KL. MR imaging of the Achilles tendon: overlap of findings in symptomatic and asymptomatic individuals. Skeletal Radiol 2000;29(11):640–5.
88. Soila K, Karjalainen PT, Aronen HJ, Pihlajamaki HK, Tirman PJ. High-resolution MR imaging of the asymptomatic Achilles tendon: new observations. AJR Am J Roentgenol 1999;173(2):323–8.
89. Saltzman CL, Tearse DS. Achilles tendon injuries. J Am Acad Orthop Surg 1998;6(5):316–25.
90. Rivenburgh DW. Physical modalities in the treatment of tendon injuries. Clin Sports Med 1992;11(3):645–59.
91. Siebert W. What is the efficacy of 'soft' and 'mid' lasers in therapy of tendinopathies? A double blind study. Arch Orthop Trauma Surg 1987;106:358–63.
92. Glass JM, Stephen RL, Jacobson SC. The quantity and distribution of radiolabeled dexamethasone delivered to tissue by iontophoresis. Int J Dermatol 1980;19(9):519–25.
93. Nowicki KD, Hummer CD 3rd, Heidt RS Jr, Colosimo AJ. Effects of iontophoretic versus injection administration of dexamethasone. Med Sci Sports Exerc 2002;34(8):1294–301.
94. Gill SS, Gelbke MK, Mattson SL, Anderson MW, Hurwitz SR. Fluoroscopically guided low-volume peritendinous corticosteroid injection for Achilles tendinopathy. A safety study. J Bone Joint Surg [Am] 2004;86A(4):802–6.
95. Neeter C, Thomee R, Silbernagel KG, Thomee P, Karlsson J. Iontophoresis with or without dexamethazone in the treatment of acute Achilles tendon pain. Scand J Med Sci Sports 2003;13(6):376–82.
96. Ozgocmen S, Kiris A, Ardicoglu O, Kocakoc E, Kaya A. Glucocorticoid iontophoresis for Achilles tendon enthesitis in ankylosing spondylitis: significant response documented by power Doppler ultrasound. Rheumatol Int 2005;25(2):158–60.
97. Alfredson H. Chronic midportion Achilles tendinopathy: an update on research and treatment. Clin Sports Med 2003;22(4):727–41.
98. Alfredson H, Lorentzon R. Chronic Achilles tendinosis: recommendations for treatment and prevention. Sports Med 2000;29(2):135–46.
99. Silbernagel KG, Thomee R, Thomee P, Karlsson J. Eccentric overload training for patients with chronic Achilles tendon pain—a randomised controlled study with reliability testing of the evaluation methods. Scand J Med Sci Sports 2001;11(4):197–206.
100. Bruckner P, Khan K. Clinical Sports Medicine, 2nd ed. Sydney: McGraw-Hill, 2001.
101. Akizuki KH, Gartman EJ, Nisonson B, Ben-Avi S, McHugh MP. The relative stress on the Achilles tendon during ambulation in an ankle immobiliser: implications for rehabilitation after Achilles tendon repair. Br J Sports Med 2001;35(5):329–33; discussion 33–4.
102. Brody. Running injuries. Prevention and management. Clin Symp 1987;39:1–36.
103. Morelli V, James E. Achilles tendonopathy and tendon rupture: conservative versus surgical management. Prim Care 2004;31(4):1039–54, x.
104. Welsh RP, Clodman J. Clinical survey of Achilles tendinitis in athletes. Can Med Assoc J 1980;122(2):193–5.
105. Appell HJ. Skeletal muscle atrophy during immobilization. Int J Sports Med 1986;7(1):1–5.
106. Astrom M, Westlin N. No effect of piroxicam on Achilles tendinopathy. A randomized study of 70 patients. Acta Orthop Scand 1992;63(6):631–4.
107. Li Z, Yang G, Khan M, Stone D, Woo SL, Wang JH. Inflammatory response of human tendon fibroblasts to cyclic mechanical stretching. Am J Sports Med 2004;32(2):435–40.

108. Fredberg U, Bolvig L, Pfeiffer-Jensen M, Clemmensen D, Jakobsen BW, Stengaard-Pedersen K. Ultrasonography as a tool for diagnosis, guidance of local steroid injection and, together with pressure algometry, monitoring of the treatment of athletes with chronic jumper's knee and Achilles tendinitis: a randomized, double-blind, placebo-controlled study. Scand J Rheumatol 2004;33(2):94–101.

109. Kapetanos G. The effect of the local corticosteroids on the healing and biomechanical properties of the partially injured tendon. Clin Orthop Rel Res 1982(163):170–9.

110. Fredberg U. Local corticosteroid injection in sport: review of literature and guidelines for treatment. Scand J Med Sci Sports 1997;7(3):131–9.

111. Shrier I, Matheson GO, Kohl HW, 3rd. Achilles tendonitis: are corticosteroid injections useful or harmful? Clin J Sport Med 1996;6(4):245–50.

112. Speed CA. Fortnightly review: Corticosteroid injections in tendon lesions. BMJ 2001;323(7309):382–6.

113. Speed C. Corticosteroid injections in tendon lesions. BMJ 2001;323(7309):382–6.

114. Astrom M. Partial rupture in chronic Achilles tendinopathy. A retrospective analysis of 342 cases. Acta Orthop Scand 1998;69(4):404–7.

115. Ljungqvist R. Subcutaneous partial rupture of the Achilles tendon. Acta Orthop Scand 1967;suppl 113:1.

116. Capasso NM. Preliminary results with peritendinous protease inhibitor injections in the management of Achilles tendinitis. J Sports Traumatol Rel Res 1993;15:37–43.

117. Tuncay I, Ozbek H, Atik B, Ozen S, Akpinar F. Effects of hyaluronic acid on postoperative adhesion of tendo calcaneus surgery: an experimental study in rats. J Foot Ankle Surg 2002;41(2):104–8.

118. Tatari H, Skiak E, Destan H, Ulukus C, Ozer E, Satoglu S. Effect of hylan G-F 20 in Achilles' tendonitis: an experimental study in rats. Arch Phys Med Rehabil 2004;85(9):1470–4.

119. Murrell GA. Using nitric oxide to treat tendinopathy. Br J Sports Med 2007;41(4):227–31.

120. Szomor ZL, Appleyard RC, Murrell GA. Overexpression of nitric oxide synthases in tendon overuse. J Orthop Res 2006;24(1):80–6.

121. Paoloni JA, Appleyard RC, Nelson J, Murrell GA. Topical nitric oxide application in the treatment of chronic extensor tendinosis at the elbow: a randomized, double-blinded, placebo-controlled clinical trial. Am J Sports Med 2003;31(6):915–20.

122. Paoloni JA, Appleyard RC, Nelson J, Murrell GA. Topical glyceryl trinitrate treatment of chronic noninsertional Achilles tendinopathy. A randomized, double-blind, placebo-controlled trial. J Bone Joint Surg [Am] 2004;86–A(5):916–22.

123. Paoloni JA, Murrell GA. Three-year followup study of topical glyceryl trinitrate treatment of chronic noninsertional Achilles tendinopathy. Foot Ankle Int 2007;28(10):1064–8.

124. Strauch B, Patel MK, Rosen DJ, Mahadevia S, Brindzei N, Pilla AA. Pulsed magnetic field therapy increases tensile strength in a rat Achilles' tendon repair model. J Hand Surg [Am] 2006;31(7):1131–5.

125. Lee EW, Maffulli N, Li CK, Chan KM. Pulsed magnetic and electromagnetic fields in experimental Achilles tendonitis in the rat: a prospective randomized study. Arch Phys Med Rehabil 1997;78(4):399–404.

126. Owoeye I, Spielholz NI, Fetto J, Nelson AJ. Low-intensity pulsed galvanic current and the healing of tenotomized rat Achilles tendons: preliminary report using load-to-breaking measurements. Arch Phys Med Rehabil 1987;68(7):415–8.

127. Vulpiani MC VM, Savoia V, Di Pangrazio E, Trischitta D, Ferretti A. Jumper's knee treatment with extracorporeal shock wave therapy: a long-term follow-up observational study. J Sports Med Phys Fitness 2007;47(3):323–8.

128. Albert JD, Meadeb J, Guggenbuhl P, . High-energy extracorporeal shock-wave therapy for calcifying tendinitis of the rotator cuff: a randomised trial. J Bone Joint Surg Br 2007;89(3):335–41.

129. Wang CJ, Ko JY, Chan YS, Weng LH, Hsu SL. Extracorporeal shockwave for chronic patellar tendinopathy. Am J Sports Med 2007;35(6):972–8.

130. Furia J. High-energy extracorporeal shock wave therapy as a treatment for insertional Achilles tendinopathy. Am J Sports Med 2006;34(5):733–40.

131. Sems A DR, Iannotti JP. Extracorporeal shock wave therapy in the treatment of chronic tendinopathies. J Am Acad Orthop Surg 2006;14(4):195–204.

132. Furia J. High-energy extracorporeal shock wave therapy as a treatment for chronic noninsertional Achilles tendinopathy. Am J Sports Med 2008;36(3):502–8.

133. Chen YJ, Wang CJ, Yang KD, et al. Extracorporeal shock waves promote healing of collagenase-induced Achilles tendinitis and increase TGF-beta1 and IGF-I expression. J Orthop Res 2004;22(4):854–61.

134. Rompe JD. Shock wave therapy for chronic Achilles tendon pain: a randomized placebo-controlled trial. Clin Orthop Rel Res 2006;445:276–7; author reply 277.

14

Nonoperative Management of Achilles Tendinopathy

Justin Paoloni and George A.C. Murrell

Anatomy

The soleus and gastrocnemius muscles combine in the calf to form the Achilles tendon, which inserts onto the posterior process of the calcaneus. The Achilles musculotendinous unit is the primary ankle plantar flexor. The Achilles tendon is the largest and strongest tendon in the body, and is able to accept weight-bearing forces of ten times body weight.[1]

The Achilles tendon has a spiral configuration, internally rotating prior to inserting inferiorly onto the posterior calcaneus. The retrocalcaneal bursa lies anterior to the Achilles tendon, is located between the tendon and the calcaneus immediately proximal to its insertion, and provides lubrication for the tendon passing over the bone. The retro-Achilles bursa is posterior to the Achilles tendon at its insertion and functions to lubricate motion between the Achilles tendon and the overlying skin. In insertional Achilles tendinopathy, both the retrocalcaneal bursa and calcaneal tuberosity, and also the retro-Achilles bursa, are potentially involved in the pathologic process.[2]

Biomechanics

During the stance phase of walking, the ankle plantar flexor muscles are dominant, and large forces act on the Achilles. Running surfaces such as hills or cambers, changes in training intensity or mileage, and inadequate footwear are proposed causes for Achilles tendinopathy.[3–5]

As the Achilles tendon inserts into the calcaneus, talocalcaneal (subtalar) motion causes tendon-shearing forces, and thus functional subtalar hyperpronation may be an etiologic factor in Achilles tendinopathy.[6,7] Subtalar pronation causes tibial internal rotation while knee extension causes tibial external rotation, and this tendon "whipping action" may compromise tendon vascularity and lead to collagen fiber degeneration.

J.A. Nunley (ed.), *The Achilles Tendon: Treatment and Rehabilitation*,
DOI: 10.1007/978-1-387-79206-4_14, © Springer Science+Business Media, LLC 2009

Pathophysiology

Achilles tendinopathy is a degenerative tendinopathy[8,9] that has an incidence in runners of 6.5% to 18%,[1,3,5] and it is suggested that a combination of anatomic and biomechanical factors cause tendon substance degeneration.[3-7,10,11]

In Achilles tendon injury, metabolic changes in the paratenon result in increased catabolism, decreased oxygenation, and impairment of paratenon gliding function.[8,9,12] The early paratenon injury probably leads to subsequent tendon substance degeneration and tendinopathy. The tendon substance degeneration may also occur as a result of tenocyte apoptosis due to repetitive loading.[13]

Histopathologically, the features of degenerative tendinopathy include collagen fiber disorganization and disruption, mucoid degeneration, neovascularization, and an absence of inflammatory cells.[8,9,14]

Animal tendon metabolism is relatively sluggish, as evidenced by its having only 13% of the oxygen uptake of muscle, and requiring more than 100 days to synthesize structurally and biomechanically mature collagen.[15] Normally, it takes 12 to 16 weeks for the development of the collagen fibers with effective cross-bonding to provide a strong elastic scar.[16] This 3- to 4-month time frame of animal tendon healing has implications for treating human tendinopathy, and this may be the reason that tendinopathies such as Achilles tendinopathy have a tendency to chronicity.

Classification

Achilles tendinopathy is classified as insertional or noninsertional. Noninsertional tendinopathy is tendon substance degeneration in the relatively hypovascular region of the Achilles tendon that is 2 to 6 cm proximal to the calcaneal insertion.[17] Insertional tendinopathy involves the tendon–bone interface and may be associated with a prominent posterosuperior calcaneal tuberosity (Haglund's deformity).[2] Haglund's deformity contributes to the development of insertional tendinopathy through mechanical abrasion and chemical erosion of the retrocalcaneal bursa and overlying tendon. The retro-Achilles bursa may also be involved in the pathologic process, often as a result of friction from footwear.

Clinical Features

The dominant symptom of Achilles tendinopathy is tendon pain. The location of the Achilles tendon pain and tenderness differentiates between insertional and noninsertional Achilles tendinopathy. With noninsertional tendinopathy, pain, swelling, and tenderness are localized 2 to 6 cm proximal to the calcaneal insertion (Fig.14.1) , whereas in insertional tendinopathy the site of pain and tenderness is localized to the tendon insertion onto the calcaneus. The pain is usually worse in the morning and may be associated with morning tendon stiffness, is initially reduced with exercising the tendon, and then may recur after exercise (see Case Study, below). With disease progression the pain may become constant, even during light exercise such as walking.

Clinical examination reveals localized tendon tenderness and often tendon thickening and crepitus on palpation. Achilles tenderness may be reduced by

Fig. 14.1. The site of pain, swelling, and tenderness in noninsertional Achilles tendinopathy, commonly 2 to 6 cm from the Achilles tendon insertion

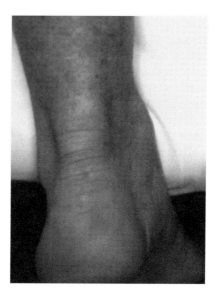

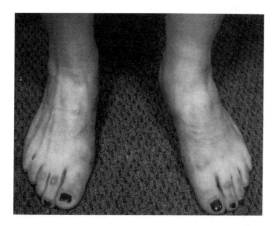

Fig. 14.2. Subtalar hyperpronation in the stance phase, most prominent in the left foot with some collapse of the medial longitudinal arch of the foot. Excessive subtalar hyperpronation may increase torsional forces on the Achilles tendon and its vasculature, and contribute to the development of Achilles tendinopathy

passive ankle dorsiflexion (London test). In insertional Achilles tendinopathy, an obvious retro-Achilles bursitis may be noted. Subtalar hyperpronation (Fig. 14.2) or pes planus may be present. Restricted ankle range of movement and clinical decreases in ankle plantarflexion strength are uncommon.

Case Study

A 42-year-old man presented with the insidious onset of 4 months of left posterior heel pain during and after running. Over the past 7 months he had increased his running distance in an effort to lose weight, and had progressed from running on a treadmill twice a week to road running four times a week. He said that he had morning pain and stiffness in the Achilles, and Achilles tendon stiffness after inactivity.

On examination it was noted that he had pes planus and subtalar hyperpronation while standing, and there was posterior heel pain with weight-bearing ankle inversion and eversion. Tenderness was present 3 to 5 cm proximal to the Achilles tendon insertion, and there was decreased tenderness in this region when the tendon was placed under passive stretch (London test).

The ankle x-ray was normal, but ultrasound demonstrated a fusiform thickening in the Achilles tendon with hypoechoic regions and collagen fiber disorganization and disruption.

Clinically and radiologically, the patient had noninsertional Achilles tendinopathy, and treatment included regular ice application, paracetamol/acetaminophen as required for pain, avoidance of aggravating activities in the short term, regular Achilles stretching, and an eccentric Achilles strengthening program. Other measures such as foot control through supportive shoes and orthotics were emphasized.

The patient presented 4 weeks later with moderate improvement in his Achilles pain, but he still had morning pain and stiffness, and stiffness after inactivity. Walking was pain free. Tenderness persisted in the Achilles tendon on examination. Orthotics were prescribed, and he was directed to wear them and his supportive footwear at all times. He was encouraged to continue the stretching and exercise program, and 1.25 mg/24-hour topical glyceryl trinitrate patches were commenced.

On review 4 weeks later, he had been compliant with all of his nonoperative treatment measures. The Achilles was virtually asymptomatic except for mild morning stiffness. Mild Achilles tenderness persisted on examination. Again, he was encouraged to continue the exercise program, wear his supportive shoes and orthotics, and use the topical glyceryl trinitrate patches.

At a further review 4 weeks later, a total of 12 weeks after commencing therapy, he had been asymptomatic for the past 2 to 3 weeks. A graded return to running was implemented, which entailed gradually reintroducing running, having rest days from activity, and wearing supportive shoes when running. He was told to continue his stretches and exercises for a further 6 to 8 weeks.

At the 16-week review he was asymptomatic and had returned to running 2 to 3 km three times a week without symptoms. He was advised to slowly increase his running and to continue maintenance stretching and exercise.

Investigations

Achilles tendinopathy is a clinical diagnosis. Weight-bearing ankle x-rays can be used to exclude bony pathology. Ultrasound (Fig.14.3) and magnetic resonance imaging (MRI) (Fig.14.4) demonstrate pathology, but are generally unnecessary. There is a high incidence of asymptomatic Achilles tendon degeneration seen with both ultrasound and MRI scans that may confound the diagnosis.[18–20]

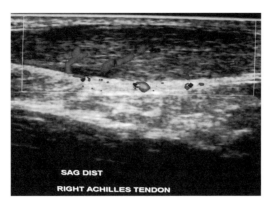

Fig. 14.3. Doppler ultrasound scan demonstrating noninsertional Achilles tendinopathy, with fusiform tendon thickening, hypoechoic regions, and increased tendon blood flow suggestive of neovascularization on Doppler mode

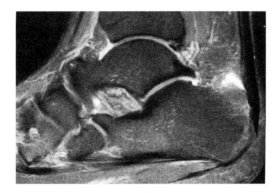

Fig. 14.4. Magnetic resonance imaging (MRI) demonstrating insertional Achilles tendinopathy with retrocalcaneal bursitis and Haglund's bony deformity of the posterior calcaneal process

Treatment

Exercise rehabilitation is the mainstay of treatment for Achilles tendinopathy.[4,10,11,21,22] There are many other suggested treatment approaches, but exercise rehabilitation has the best evidence of efficacy, and should be at the core of any treatment program.

Resting from aggravating activities (relative rest or activity modification) is logical, but lacks evidence of clinical efficacy. However, given that it is generally accepted that Achilles tendon degeneration results from overuse or overload, and that the time frame for tendon healing is probably 3 to 4 months, it is reasonable to instruct the patient to avoid aggravating activities in the short term. If the patient is unable to rest, or has severe pain, a plaster boot with a rocker-bottom sole is advocated for 6 weeks to enforce relative rest.[4]

Analgesics may be required for the pain of Achilles tendinopathy and, initially, regular ice application should be encouraged as a simple measure of controlling tendon pain and swelling. Paracetamol/acetaminophen/Tylenol is as effective as nonsteroidal antiinflammatory drugs (NSAIDs) for analgesia in soft tissue injury,[23,24] and NSAIDs have not demonstrated clinical efficacy in treating Achilles tendinopathy.[25–27] Thus, if analgesia is required in Achilles tendinopathy, paracetamol/acetaminophen is probably the best choice. In bursitis associated with insertional Achilles tendinopathy, NSAIDs may be appropriate for analgesia.

Heel lift devices reduce Achilles tendon plantarflexion stresses during walking [28] and are an inexpensive treatment modality. It is suggested that these 1.5-cm heel lifts be used bilaterally in all shoes.[4] Orthotic devices can control subtalar motion in patients with subtalar hyperpronation, and have been advocated to reduce Achilles tendon stress during weight-bearing activities such as walking or running.[4,6,7,29–32]

Stretching the Achilles tendon restores tendon length and stimulates tendon healing along the lines of normal force loading.[33,34] While stretching has limited evidence of clinical efficacy in treating Achilles tendinopathy, basic science research suggests that stretching assists in the restoration of normal biomechanical properties of an injured tendon. Prolonged static stretching of both the gastrocnemius and soleus muscles (with straight knee and with bent knee stretches, respectively) is therefore advocated as part of the treatment program.

Eccentric Achilles tendon exercises such as heel-drop exercises off a step (Fig.14.5) decrease pain and hasten the return to normal activity in patients with chronic noninsertional Achilles tendinopathy when performed at high repetitions for 12 weeks (Alfredson protocol).[35] Concentric heel raises to return to the neutral ankle position are not performed on the affected leg with

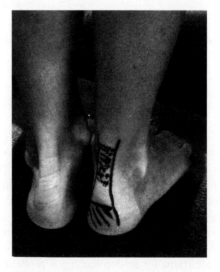

Fig. 14.5. Eccentric Achilles tendon strengthening exercises as per the Alfredson protocol. These exercises are often described as "heel-drop" exercises and are performed with the forefoot on the step and the hindfoot hanging off the edge of the step in order to lower the heel below the level of the step. This lowering of the heel causes Achilles tendon lengthening under load, and this eccentric exercise stimulates tendon healing. Note that there is no concentric component to the exercises

this exercise regime, as they decrease efficacy.[36] Eccentric exercise used in the treatment of insertional Achilles tendinopathy appears to be less effective,[37] and early in the course of treatment stretching or exercise may increase Achilles tendon pain. It may be advisable to avoid these activities in the initial stages of treating insertional Achilles tendinopathy, and to concentrate on decreasing mechanical trauma to the tendon, and inflammation such as with concomitant bursitis.[10,24,38]

Corticosteroid injections have a demonstrated lack of efficacy in Achilles tendinopathy and peritendinitis,[39] have a risk of tendon rupture with intratendinous injection, and generally should not be used to treat noninsertional Achilles tendinopathy.[40–42] Corticosteroid injection may be used in insertional Achilles tendinopathy where concomitant bursitis is present and symptomatic.[24,41,43]

Extracorporeal shockwave therapy (ESWT) has shown efficacy in treating recalcitrant insertional Achilles tendinopathy,[44] and recently has shown treatment benefits in treating noninsertional Achilles tendinopathy that are similar to eccentric exercise.[45] Currently, ESWT is probably best reserved for treating recalcitrant Achilles tendinopathy.

Continuous topical glyceryl trinitrate treatment at a dosage of 1.25 mg/24 hours has demonstrated efficacy in improving asymptomatic patient outcomes in chronic noninsertional Achilles tendinopathy when combined with exercise rehabilitation,[46] and these effects persist at the 3-year follow-up [47](Fig.14.6) . This therapy is best used in chronic noninsertional Achilles tendinopathy if the initial treatment is ineffective, and it should be recognized that this drug has not been approved for this purpose by the Food and Drug Administration (FDA) at the time of publication. Side effects include headache and rash in 5% to 10% of patients. The efficacy in treating insertional Achilles tendinopathy is not established.

Aprotinin, a metalloprotease and collagenase inhibitor, has limited evidence of efficacy in decreasing tendon pain and improving functional outcomes in Achilles tendinopathy,[48] with recent research suggesting it is no more effective than a placebo.[49]

The most common side effect is a mild allergic reaction in 3% of patients, although anaphylactic reaction can occur. Aprotinin injections are probably

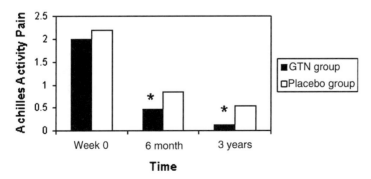

Fig. 14.6. Graph illustrating the effects of continuous topical glyceryl trinitrate (GTN) treatment on Achilles tendon pain with activity in patients with chronic noninsertional Achilles tendinopathy. Significant differences at the *p* <.05 level are denoted by an asterisk

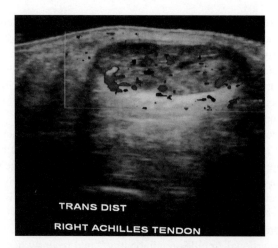

Fig. 14.7. Cross-sectional view of the Achilles tendon with Doppler ultrasound demonstrating increased blood flow within the tendon substance, suggestive of neovascularization in tendinopathy. Note that the majority of increased blood flow is in the deep aspect of the tendon. This neovascularization can be obliterated using polidocinol sclerosant injections, similar to the process of treating varicose veins, and provides 80% pain reduction in 80% of people over 4 to 6 months

best reserved for recalcitrant tendinopathy due to the risk of anaphylaxis, and it should be recognized that this drug had not been approved for this purpose by the FDA at the time of publication.

Doppler ultrasound-guided polidocinol injections, a sclerosant agent used to obliterate regions of neovascularization in tendinopathy (Fig.14.7) , has evidence of efficacy in decreasing pain and improving patient outcomes in Achilles tendinopathy,[50,51] and this effect persists at 2-year follow-up.[52] This therapy has no side effects, but it is relatively new, and therefore availability is currently limited to specialized centers.

Another treatment that has been advocated for use in musculoskeletal injury such as Achilles tendinopathy is prolotherapy, the use of proliferative agents such as high-strength glucose, although there is no evidence of efficacy in treating any tendon injury.[24,53] The use of prolotherapy in Achilles tendinopathy would generally be considered a last resort.

With any tendinopathy, including Achilles tendinopathy, failure of symptom resolution with 6 to 12 months of nonoperative treatment may indicate the necessity for surgical intervention. The presence of unacceptable pain or disability from the patient's perspective should prompt orthopedic surgical referral.

Return to Sports

In Achilles tendinopathy, return to full sports activity is variable, but may take as long as 6 to 12 months. Cross-training to maintain fitness and control body weight should be encouraged and will generally involve pain-free, non–weight-bearing activities such as cycling, swimming, or rowing. Once the patient is asymptomatic with daily activities such as walking, then a graded return to more vigorous weight-bearing activities, such as walking for exercise or running, may be instituted. This return to heavy weight-bearing activity should always be performed gradually with an emphasis on wearing supportive footwear to control excessive foot motion, ensuring rest days to allow for tendon adaptation to increased stress, and monitoring Achilles symptoms to prevent overload and injury recurrence.

Prognosis

One of the few studies of the natural course of Achilles tendinopathy was an 8-year follow-up study to determine the long-term outcome of patients initially treated nonoperatively for acute or subacute Achilles tendinopathy.[54] This study demonstrated that the long-term prognosis of patients with Achilles tendinopathy was generally good, with 94% of people being asymptomatic or with only mild Achilles tendon pain on strenuous exercise, and 84% of people returning to full levels of physical activity. Despite these encouraging outcomes, there was a clear side-to-side difference between the involved and the uninvolved Achilles tendon in the performance tests, clinical examination, and ultrasonography, and 29% of patients with Achilles tendinopathy failed to respond to nonoperative treatment and required surgical treatment.

References

1. Clain M, Baxter D.E. Achilles tendinitis. Foot Ankle Int 1992 ;13(8): 482–7.
2. Merkel K, Hess H, Kunz M. Insertional tendinopathy in athletes: a light microscope, histochemical and electron microscope examination. Pathol Res Pract 1982;173:303–9.
3. Clement D, Taunton JE, Smart GW. A survey of overuse running injuries. Physician Sports Med 1981;9(5):47–58.
4. Brukner P, Khan K. Clinical Sports Medicine, 3rd ed. Sydney: Blackwell Scientific, 2005.
5. Krissoff W, Ferris WD. Runner's injuries. Physician Sports Med 1979;7(12):55–64.
6. Burdett R. Forces predicted at the ankle during running. Med Sci Sports 1982;14: 308–16.
7. Scott S, Winter DA. Internal forces at chronic running injury sites. Med Sci Sports Exerc 1990;22(3):357–69.
8. Khan K, Cook JL, Bonar F, . Histopathology of common tendinopathies. Sports Med 1999;27(6):393–408.
9. Astrom M, Rausing A. Chronic Achilles tendinopathy: a survey of surgical and histopathological findings. Clin Orthop 1995;316:151–64.
10. Alfredson H, Lorentzon R. Chronic Achilles tendinosis. Recommendations for treatment and prevention. Sports Med 2000;29(2):135–46.
11. Renstrom AFH. An introduction to chronic overuse injuries. In: Harris M, Williams C, Stanish WD eds., ., Oxford Textbook of Sports Medicine. New York: Oxford University Press, 1994:531–45.
12. Kvist M, Jozsa L, Jarvinen M. Chronic Achilles paratenonitis in athletes: a histological and histochemical study. Pathology 1987;19:1–11.
13. Arnoczky S, Tian T, Lavagnino M, . Activation of stress-activated protein kinases (SAPK) in tendon cells following cyclic strain: the effects of strain frequency, strain magnitude, and cytosolic calcium. J Orthop Res 2002;20:947–52.
14. Puddu G, Ippolito E, Postacchini F. A classification of Achilles tendon disease. Am J Sports Med 1976;4:145–50.

15. Murrell G, Jang D, Deng XH, . Effects of exercise on Achilles tendon healing in a rat model. Foot Ankle Int 1998;19(9):598–603.
16. Vailas A, Tipton CM, Laughlin HL, . Physical activity and hypophysectomy on the aerobic capacity of ligaments and tendons. J Appl Physiol 1978;44(4):542–6.
17. Lagergen C. Vascular distribution in Achilles tendon—an angiographic and micro-angiographic study. Acta Chir Scand 1958;116:491–5.
18. Harris CA, Peduto AJ. Achilles tendon imaging. Aust Radiol 2006;50(6):513–25.
19. Cook JL, Khan KM, Purdam C. Achilles tendinopathy. Manual Ther 2002;7(3):121–30.
20. Kainberger F, Mittermaier F, Seidl G, . Imaging of tendons-adaptation, degeneration, rupture. Eur J Radiol 1997;25(3):209–22.
21. Werd MB. Achilles tendon sports injuries: a review of classification and treatment. J Am Podiatr Med Assoc 2007;97(1):37–48.
22. McLauchlan GJ, Handoll HH. Interventions for treating acute and chronic Achilles tendinitis. Cochrane Data System Rev 2001;2.
23. DeGara C, Taylor M, Hedges A. Assessment of analgesic drugs in soft tissue injuries presenting to an accident and emergency department—a comparison of antrafenine, paracetamol, and placebo. Postgrad Med J 1982;58:489–92.
24. Paoloni JA, Orchard J. The use of therapeutic medications in soft tissue injuries. Med J Aust 2005;183(7):384–8.
25. McLauchlan G, Handoll HHG. Interventions for treating acute and chronic Achilles tendinitis. Cochrane Data System Rev 2004;4.
26. Astrom M, Westlin N. No effect of piroxicam on Achilles tendinopathy. A randomized study of 70 patients. Acta Orthop Scand 1992;63(6):631–4.
27. Auclair J, Georges M, Grapton X, . A double-blind controlled multicenter study of percutaneous niflumic acid gel and placebo in the treatment of Achilles heel tendinitis. Curr Ther Res Clin Exp 1989;46(4):782–8.
28. Akizuki KH, Gartman EJ, Nisonson B, . The relative stress on the Achilles tendon during ambulation in an ankle immobiliser: implications for rehabilitation after Achilles tendon repair. Br J Sports Med 2001;35(5):329–33.
29. Wilson JJ, Best TM. Common overuse tendon problems: a review and recommendations for treatment. Am Fam Phys 2005;72(5):811–8.
30. Wallace RG, Traynor IE, Kernohan WG, . Combined conservative and orthotic management of acute ruptures of the Achilles tendon. J Bone Joint Surg [Am] 2004;86–A(6):1198–202.
31. Mazzone MF, McCue T. Common conditions of the Achilles tendon. Am Fam Phys 2002;65(9):1805–10.
32. Sobel E, Levitz SJ, Caselli MA. Orthoses in the treatment of rear foot problems. J Am Podiatr Med Assoc 1999;89(5):220–33.
33. Iwuagwu F, McGrouther DA. Early cellular response in tendon injury: the effect of loading. Plast Recon Surg 1998;102(6):2064–71.
34. Kvist M, Jarvinen M. Clinical, histochemical and biomechanical features in repair of muscle and tendon injuries. Int J Sports Med 1982;3:12–14.
35. Alfredson H, Pietila T, Jonsson P, . Heavy-load eccentric calf muscle training for the treatment of chronic Achilles tendinosis. Am J Sports Med 1998;26(3):360–6.
36. Niesen-Vertommen S, Taunton JE, Clement DB. The effect of eccentric versus concentric exercise in the management of Achilles tendonitis. Clin J Sports Med 1992;2:109–13.
37. Fahlstrom M, Jonsson P, Lorentzon R, . Chronic Achilles tendon pain treated with eccentric calf-muscle training. Knee Surg Sports Traumatol Arth 2003;11(5):327–33.
38. Krishna Sayana M, Maffulli N. Insertional Achilles tendinopathy. Foot Ankle Clin 2005;10(2):309–20.
39. DaCruz DJ, Geeson M, Allen MJ, . Achilles paratendonitis: an evaluation of steroid injection. Br J Sports Med 1988;22(2):64–5.

40. Kennedy J, Willis RB. The effects of local steroid injections on tendons: a biome-chanical and microscopic correlative study. Am J Sports Med 1976;4:11–21.
41. Hayes DW Jr, Gilbertson EK, Mandracchia VJ, . Tendon pathology in the foot. The use of corticosteroid injection therapy. Clin Podiatr Med Surg 2000;17(4):723–35.
41. Shrier I, Matheson GO, Kohl HW 3rd. Achilles tendonitis: are corticosteroid injec-tions useful or harmful? Clin J Sport Med 1996;6(4):245–50.
42. Speed CA. Fortnightly review: corticosteroid injections in tendon lesions. Br Med J 2001;323(7309):382–6.
43. Furia JP. High-energy extracorporeal shock wave therapy as a treatment for inser-tional Achilles tendinopathy. Am J Sports Med 2006;34(5):733–40.
44. Rompe JD, Nafe B, Furia JP, . Eccentric loading, shock-wave treatment, or a wait-and-see policy for tendinopathy of the main body of tendo Achillis: a randomized controlled trial. Am J Sports Med 2007;35(3):374–83.
45. Paoloni JA, Appleyard RC, Nelson J, Topical glyceryl trinitrate application in the treatment of non-insertional Achilles tendinopathy: a randomized, double-blind, placebo controlled clinical trial. J Bone Joint Surg 2004;86A(5):916–22.
46. Paoloni J and Murrell GAC. Three-year prospective comparison study of topical glyceryl trinitrate treatment in chronic noninsertional Achilles tendinopathy. Foot Ankle Int 2007;28:1064–8.
47. Capasso G, Maffulli N, Testa V. Preliminary results with peritendinous protease inhibitor injections in the management of Achilles tendinitis. J Sports Traumatol Rel Res 1993;15:37–40.
48. Brown R, Orchard J, Kinchington M, . Aprotinin in the management of Achilles tendinopathy: a randomised controlled trial. Br J Sports Med 2006;40(3):275–9.
49. Alfredson H, Ohberg L. Sclerosing injections to areas of neo-vascularisation reduce pain in chronic Achilles tendinopathy: a double-blind randomised control-led trial. Knee Surg Sports Traumatol Arth 2005;13(4):338–44.
50. Alfredson H, Lorentzon R. Sclerosing polidocanol injections of small vessels to treat the chronic painful tendon. Cardio Hematol Agents Med Chem 2007;5(2):97–100.
51. Lind B, Ohberg L, Alfredson H. Sclerosing polidocanol injections in mid-portion Achilles tendinosis: remaining good clinical results and decreased tendon thickness at 2–year follow-up. Knee Surg Sports Traumatol Arth 2006;14(12):1327–32.
52. Rabago D, Best TM, Beamsley M, . A systematic review of prolotherapy for chronic musculoskeletal pain. Clin J Sport Med 2005;15(5):376–80.
53. Paavola M, Kannus P, Paakkala T, . Long-term prognosis of patients with Achilles tendinopathy: an observational 8-year follow-up study. Am J Sports Med 2000;28(5): 634–42.

15

Surgical Management of Achilles Tendinopathy by Percutaneous Longitudinal Tenotomies

Ansar Mahmood and Nicola Maffulli

Achilles tendinopathy is common among athletes, particularly those involved in very strenuous and sudden takeoff maneuvers during their sport. This includes participants in racquet sports, track and field, volleyball, and soccer.[1] Due to greater participation in recreational and competitive sporting activities, the incidence of Achilles tendinopathy has recently increased (see Case Study, below). However, Achilles tendinopathy does not exclusively affect athletes. Health professionals in both primary and secondary care are increasingly consulted by patients suffering from Achilles tendinopathy. Familiarity with the management options is important to best advise individual patients.

The management of Achilles tendinopathy lacks evidence-based support, and sufferers of the condition are at risk of long-term morbidity with often unpredictable clinical outcomes.[2] A substantial number of working days is lost annually due to Achilles tendinopathy. [3]

Case Study

A 26-year-old male tennis player was referred to our orthopedic foot and ankle clinic with a history of pain and discomfort around the region of his Achilles tendon and posterior ankle for the previous 6 months. The discomfort was relieved initially by gentle exercise, but then became worse after a game of tennis. There was associated swelling on occasion, and he had modified the way that he walked up and down stairs. The patient had some physiotherapy initiated by his primary care physician, but felt that the benefit from it had reached a plateau. He still had residual pain and discomfort. He was otherwise systemically well with no medical comorbidities or allergies.

On examination, the patient walked without a limp, and was able to stand on tiptoes with mild discomfort. This excluded rupture of the Achilles tendon. Further examination was conducted with the patient prone. The patient was tender on palpation over the Achilles tendon, with maximal tenderness about

J.A. Nunley (ed.), *The Achilles Tendon: Treatment and Rehabilitation*,
DOI: 10.1007/978-1-387-79206-4_15, © Springer Science+Business Media, LLC 2009

3 cm proximal to the insertion of the Achilles tendon onto the calcaneum. This area felt thickened in relation to the adjacent tendon. There was no readily visible swelling or skin changes. The Simmonds/Thompson[4] and Matles[5] tests were negative, confirming that a rupture was not present. The painful arc sign was positive; the area of thickening moved in relation to the malleoli when the foot was moved passively from full dorsiflexion to plantarflexion.[6] This indicated an intratendinous rather than a paratendinous pathology. The tenderness in this area diminished significantly on applying tension to the tendon, with ankle dorsiflexion. This is known as the Royal London test, and is highly specific (91%) for Achilles tendinopathy.[7]

Achilles tendinopathy is usually established as the diagnosis from a detailed history and focused examination. However, if the diagnosis is unclear, then imaging can be used to confirm the clinical suspicion. Ultrasound is often used primarily. Although considered operator-dependent, both ultrasound scanning and magnetic resonance imaging (MRI), in the right hands, show intratendinous morphology and pathology, allowing better understanding of the condition.

Symptoms

Classic Patient History and Findings

Patients complain of burning pain in the posterior aspect of the calf and ankle, often worse at the beginning of a training session and after exercise. Some patients have difficulty taking the first few steps in the morning. In severe cases, there may be pain during activities of daily living, including walking and stair climbing. The degree of morning stiffness correlates well with the severity of the disease in the tendon.[8]

Clinical diagnosis is mostly based on a combination of palpation, use of the painful-arc sign, and the Royal London test. In paratendinopathy, the area of tenderness and thickening remains fixed in relation to the malleoli when the ankle is moved from full dorsiflexion into plantarflexion. If the lesion lies within the tendon, the point of tenderness and any swelling associated with it moves with the tendon as the ankle is brought from full dorsiflexion into plantarflexion. In mixed lesions, both motion and fixation of the swelling and of the tenderness can be detected in relation to the malleoli.

In the acute phase, the tendon is diffusely swollen and edematous, and on palpation tenderness is usually greatest 2 to 6 cm proximal to the tendon insertion. In paratendinopathy, fibrin precipitated from the fibrinogen-rich fluid around the tendon can cause palpable crepitation. In lesions of the main body of the tendon, a tender, nodular swelling at the site of the failed healing response is present.

Imaging

Ultrasound Scan

Ultrasound scan is a powerful diagnostic aid. An ultrasonographic diagnosis of tendinopathy can be made when the tendon presents an altered intratendinous structure—at times with a well-defined focal area of heterogeneous acoustic signal. An ultrasonographic diagnosis of paratendinopathy is made when the peritenon is thickened or shows altered echogenicity. If power Doppler is available, it shows increased vascularity around the hypoechoic area, which is thought to represent neovascularization as part of a failed healing response. This contradicts the classical teaching that tendinopathy is associated with hypovascularity.

Magnetic Resonance Imaging

Magnetic resonance imaging provides extensive information on the internal morphology of the tendon and the surrounding structures, and is useful to evaluate various stages of chronic degeneration. Excellent correlation between MRI and pathologic findings at surgery has been reported.[9]

Due to the high sensitivity of these imaging modalities, an abnormality should be interpreted with caution and correlated with the patient's symptoms before making any management recommendations.

Treatment

Conservative Management

Conservative management is recommended in the initial phases with identification and correction of possible etiologic factors, at times using a symptom-related approach.

Despite the absence of scientific evidence for an ongoing chemical inflammation inside the tendon, nonsteroidal antiinflammatory drugs (NSAIDs) are commonly used as part of the initial management. Their use to diminish chemical inflammation in the chronic painful Achilles tendon should be questioned. Indeed, in a randomized, double-blind, placebo-controlled study of 70 patients with chronic painful Achilles tendinopathy, oral piroxicam gave similar results as placebo.[10]

The use of steroids for tendinopathy is controversial, as corticosteroid injections may produce a partial rupture in patients with chronic Achilles tendinopathy.[3] Gill et al.,[11] in a retrospective cohort study, established the safety of low-volume injections of corticosteroids for the management of Achilles tendinopathy when the corticosteroids are carefully injected into the peritendinous space under direct fluoroscopic visualization. However, this is not routine practice in most centers.

Modalities such as cold therapy, heat, massage, ultrasound, electrical stimulation, and laser therapy are used. These modalities are reported to be effective, but there are very few prospective or randomized controlled trials that confirm their effects. The initial conservative management is directed toward presumed etiologic factors or toward relieving symptoms. Most commonly, it consists of a combination of strategies, including abstention from the activities that caused the symptoms, and correction of training errors, foot malalignments, decreased flexibility, and muscle weakness.[12] Complete rest of the tendon is indicated only to alleviate acute symptoms. Following this, the patient should be encouraged to load the tendon, which promotes collagen repair and remodeling. This can be done in a way to allow normal motion in the uninjured parts while only partially loading the injured segment. This modified rest was described by Alfredson and Lorentzon[12] in 2000. Rompe et al.,[13] in a randomized controlled trial, have shown that there is significant symptomatic benefit from eccentric loading and repetitive low-energy shock wave therapy in patients with chronic Achilles tendinopathy (>6 months) at 4 months follow-up.

Surgical Management

Surgery is recommended for patients in whom nonoperative management has proved ineffective for between 3 and 6 months. Of patients with Achilles tendon problems, 24% to 45.5% fail to respond to conservative management, and eventually require surgery.[14,15]

There are minor variations in surgical technique for tendinopathy. Nevertheless, the fundamental objective is to excise fibrotic adhesions, remove degenerated nodules, and make multiple longitudinal incisions in the tendon to influence the pathology of any detected intratendinous lesions. This is thought to restore well-ordered vascularity, and possibly stimulate tenocytes to initiate a cell matrix response to promote healing.[16,17] Recent investigations show that multiple longitudinal tenotomies trigger neoangiogenesis at the Achilles tendon, with increased blood flow.[18] This would result in improved nutrition and a more favorable environment for healing.

Most authors report excellent or good results in up to 85% of patients. However, this is not necessarily the case in low-volume, non-specialized practice.[19,20]

Preoperative Planning

Once the diagnosis is made, the patient's general health and comorbidities should be assessed. Although we generally perform the procedure with the patient under local anesthesia, in some patients general anesthesia may be necessary, and appropriate preparation should be made for those individuals.

The preoperative functional status should be noted. The skin quality and neurovascular status of the affected limb should be examined. And the status of the sural nerve should be documented. Patients also should have appropriate deep vein thrombosis (DVT) prophylaxis.

Valid informed consent should be obtained, and the patient should be aware of the risks of infection, bleeding, wound and scar problems, the operation's failure to relieve symptoms, and that further surgery may be required.

Open Approach

For multifocal, chronic recurrent Achilles tendinopathy and pantendinopathy, we prefer the open technique. This allows direct visualization and removal of all the pathologic segments, as well as sharp dissection and stripping of the paratenon. We have found that this gives a good result in about 85% of patients, whereas using percutaneous techniques for these situations may drop favorable results to 65%.

When an open surgical approach is necessary, we use a longitudinal curved incision, with the concave part toward the tendon centered over the abnormal part of the tendon. Placing the incision medially avoids injury to the sural nerve and short saphenous vein, and the curvature of the incision prevents direct exposure of the tendon in case of skin breakdown.

The paratenon and crural fascia are incised and dissected from the underlying tendon. If necessary, the tendon is freed from adhesions on the posterior, medial and lateral aspects. The paratenon should be excised obliquely as a transverse excision may produce a constriction ring, which may require revision surgery. Areas of thickened, fibrotic, and inflamed tendon are excised. The pathology can often be identified by the change in color and texture of the tendon. The lesions are then excised, and the defect can either be sutured in a side-to-side fashion or left open. We leave it open.

Hemostasis is ensured using pressure or bipolar diathermy. As any bleeding is directly seen and stopped, this reduces the incidence of postoperative hematoma.

Given the tenuous blood supply around the distal Achilles tendon, open procedures can lead to problems with wound healing and an increased chance of wound breakdown or infection. Hemostasis is important, since the reduction of postoperative bleeding speeds up recovery, diminishes the chance of wound infection, and diminishes any possible fibrotic inflammatory reaction.

Percutaneous Techniques

Ultrasound-Guided Percutaneous Tenotomy

The surgery is done on an outpatient basis. The patient lies prone on the examination couch with the feet protruding beyond the edge, and the ankles resting on a sandbag. A bloodless field is not necessary, and we do not use a tourniquet. The tendon is accurately palpated, and the area of maximum swelling or tenderness is marked and checked by ultrasound scanning. The skin is appropriately prepared with antiseptic, and a sterile longitudinal 7.5-MHz ultrasound probe is used to image the area of tendinopathy. Before infiltrating the skin and the subcutaneous tissues over the Achilles tendon with 10 mL of 1% lidocaine (lignocaine hydrochloride, Evans Medical Ltd., Leatherhead, England), 7 mL of the same solution is used to infiltrate the space between the tendon and the paratenon. This distends the paratenon and may assist in the breakdown of adhesions present between the tendon and the paratenon, as well as achieveing local anesthesia.

Under ultrasound control, a No. 11 surgical scalpel blade (Swann–Morton, Sheffield, England) is inserted into the center of the area of thickening or nodularity, aiming to be parallel to the long axis of the tendon fibers (Fig. 15.1) . The cutting edge of the blade points caudally, and penetrates the whole thickness of the tendon (Fig. 15.2) . While keeping the blade still, a full passive ankle flexion is produced and held (Fig. 15.3) . While in that position, the scalpel blade is then retracted to the surface of the tendon, inclined 45 degrees on the sagittal axis, and the blade is inserted medially through the original tenotomy (Fig. 15.4) . Keeping the blade still, a full passive ankle flexion is produced again.

The whole procedure is repeated, inclining the blade 45 degrees laterally to the original tenotomy, all the while using the same incision of the original tenotomy (Fig. 15.4). Keeping the blade still, a full passive ankle flexion is produced and held.

The blade is then partially retracted to the posterior surface of the Achilles tendon, reversed 180 degrees, so that its cutting edge now points cranially, and the whole procedure is repeated, taking care to dorsiflex the ankle passively (Figs. 15.5 and 15.6).

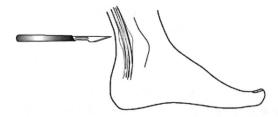

Fig. 15.1. The scalpel blade is inserted into the predetermined area of tendinopathy with the sharp edge pointing caudally

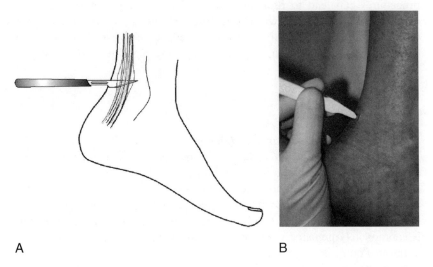

A   B

Fig. 15.2. (A,B) The scalpel blade penetrates the *whole* thickness of the Achilles tendon

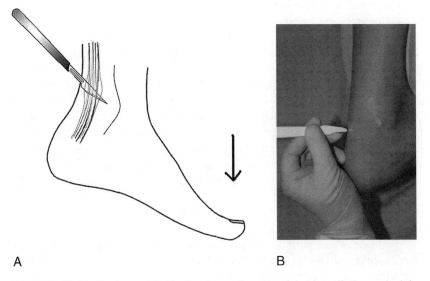

A   B

Fig.15.3. (A,B) Passive ankle flexion is produced and held until the scalpel is retracted.

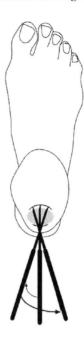

Fig. 15.4. The procedure is repeated with the blade inclined at 45 degrees medial and 45 degrees lateral to the original tenotomy

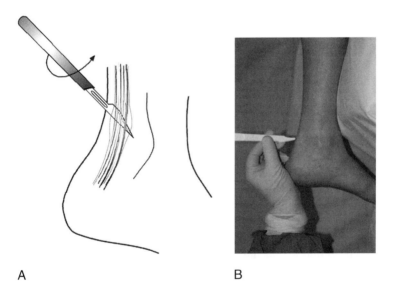

A   B

Fig. 15.5. (A,B) The blade is reversed 180 degrees to repeat the procedure on the proximal tendon

Preliminary cadaveric studies showed that a tenotomy averaging 2.8 cm long is obtained through a stab wound in the main body of the tendon.[21] A Steri-Strip (3M United Kingdom PLC, Bracknell, Berkshire, England) can be applied on the stab wound, or the stab wound can be left open. The wound is dressed with cotton swabs, and several layers of cotton wool and a crepe bandage are applied.

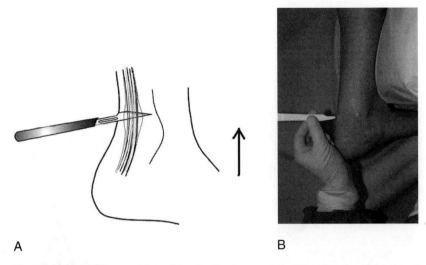

A   B

Fig. 15.6. (A,B) The sequence of tenotomies is repeated with ankle dorsiflexion and the 45 degrees medial and 45 degrees lateral inclination to the original tenotomy.

Percutaneous Multiple Longitudinal Tenotomies
The surgery is done on an outpatient basis. The patient lies prone on the operating table with the feet protruding beyond the edge. We rest the ankles on a sandbag. A bloodless field is not necessary. The figures used for the preceding technique (Figs. 15.5 and 15.6) can be used to reference this technique, as it is similar in principle with only minor variations.

The tendon is accurately palpated, and the area of maximum swelling or tenderness is marked, and checked again by ultrasound scan on the day of surgery. The skin and the subcutaneous tissues over the Achilles tendon are generously infiltrated with 15 mL of plain 1% lignocaine.

A No. 11 surgical scalpel blade is inserted parallel to the long axis of the tendon fibers in the marked area(s) with the cutting edge pointing cranially. Keeping the blade still, a full passive ankle dorsiflexion movement is produced. After reversing the position of the blade, a full passive ankle plantarflexion movement is produced. A variable area of tenolysis, in the region of about 3 cm, is thus obtained through a stab wound.

The procedure is repeated 2 cm medial and proximally, medial and distally, lateral and proximally, and lateral and distally to the site of the first stab wound.

The five wounds are closed with Steri-Strips, dressed with cotton swabs, and a few layers of cotton wool and a crepe bandage are applied.

Postoperative Care

The postoperative care regime and rehabilitation is similar for both open and percutaneous techniques.

On admission, patients are taught to perform isometric contractions of their triceps surae. Patients are instructed to perform the isometric strength training at maximum dorsiflexion, maximum plantarflexion, and at a point midway between the two.

The foot is kept elevated on the first postoperative day, and NSAIDs plus other simple analgesics are used as required for pain control. Early active dorsi- and plantarflexion of the foot are encouraged. On day 2, the patients are allowed to walk using elbow crutches, permitting partial weight-bearing as able. The bandage is reduced after 48 to 72 hours, and full weight-bearing is allowed as tolerated.

Stationary cycling and isometric, concentric, and eccentric strengthening of the calf muscles are started under physiotherapy guidance after 4 weeks. Swimming and water running are encouraged from the second week. Gentle running is started 4 to 6 weeks postoperatively, and the distance gradually increased as comfort allows. Hill workouts or interval training are allowed after a further 6 weeks. Most patients commence normal activity at around 3 months postoperatively. Patients normally discontinue physiotherapy supervision by 6 months.

Results

Ultrasound-Guided Percutaneous Tenotomy

Seventy-five athletes with unilateral Achilles tendinopathy were managed with this technique.[22] In seven patients, more than a single stab was produced due to multiple lesions or large tendinopathic lesions.

All patients were able to weight bear on the operated limb by the second postoperative day. At final review, 51 months (standard deviation [SD], 18.2) (range, 36 to 102) from the operation, 63 patients attended: 35 patients were rated excellent, 12 good, nine fair, and seven poor. Of the 16 patients in whom the procedure was not successful, eight had a pantendinopathy, 13 were runners (either middle distance or sprinters), and three were soccer players. Also, although the average interval between beginning of symptoms and operation in these patients was not significantly different from the whole group (21.6 versus 19.2 months), these patients had received more peritendinous injections (group average: 1.3; average in the patients with a fair or poor result: 2.7), and had been less compliant with their preoperative conservative management.

Nine of these 16 patients underwent a formal exploration of the Achilles tendon 7 to 12 months after the index procedure. A nodular area of tendinopathy was identified by palpation, and excised by sharp dissection. Five patients who underwent formal exploration had given up their original sport by the time of the latest review, but were able to undertake jogging and cycling.

Sixty-two subjects (83%) reported symptomatic benefits from surgery and had returned to engaging in sports. The median time to return to sports was 6.5 months (range 11 weeks to 14 months), with only two of the subjects who had returned to sports doing so after 10 months. At final follow-up, 55 of the 63 patients followed up at an average of 51 months from the operation continued to report symptomatic benefits, and 47 of 63 were still able to practice sports.

Multiple Percutaneous Longitudinal Tenotomies

The procedure was performed in 52 athletes who were training regularly, and competed up to international standards. All were able to weight bear on the operated limb by the third postoperative day.

At final review, at an average of 22.1 ± 6.5 months (range, 18 to 60) from the operation, 47 patients attended. Of these, 27 patients rated themselves as excellent, 12 as good, seven as fair, and four as poor.

Of the 11 patients in whom the procedure was not successful, two patients with a poor result and one with a fair result underwent a formal open exploration of their Achilles tendon at an average of 10 months after the original procedure. In the ones with poor results, after the peritenon was stripped through sharp dissection, a small intratendinous nodule was found in each patient and excised through a longitudinal tenotomy. The tendons were not repaired. Comparing the stab wounds with the position of the nodules, we had either missed them in the first operation or they had developed subsequently. In the patient with a fair result, a chronic paratendinopathy with fibrous peritendinous adhesions was found. The tendon was freed by sharp dissection.

In all but one of the 11 patients with a fair and poor result, the tendinopathy was associated with paratendinopathy. The three patients who underwent formal exploration resumed their sports after the open procedure. Of the remaining eight patients, five patients gave up their sport, and three were able to undertake occasional jogging.

Complications

Ultrasound-Guided Percutaneous Tenotomy

Five patients developed a subcutaneous hematoma. All such hematomas resolved with a pressure bandage, which was removed 3 to 7 days later. In another patient, a superficial infection developed 1 week after the procedure and was treated by oral antibiotic for 1 week; recovery was uneventful. At the 6-week follow-up appointment, eight patients complained of hypersensitivity of their scars when kneeling down. They were counselled to rub hand cream over their scars several times a day, and became asymptomatic 3 to 6 weeks later.

No hypertrophic or keloid scars were noted at the latest follow-up. Cosmesis was acceptable to every patient.

Eleven patients complained of morning stiffness of the ankle in the early postoperative period, but they did not report the complaint at the 6-month evaluation.

Multiple Percutaneous Longitudinal Tenotomies

Four patients developed a subcutaneous hematoma, and one patient suffered from a superficial infection of one of the stab wounds. This was treated by oral antibiotics for 5 days, and healed uneventfully. Three patients complained of hypersensitivity of the stab wounds. They were counselled to rub hand cream over their stab wounds several times a day, and were asymptomatic by the sixth postoperative week.

One patient developed a hypertrophic painful scar of three of the five stab wounds. These were injected with corticosteroids, and the patient reported a good functional and cosmetic result. At final review, only three patients were not pleased with the cosmesis of their operation scars.

References

1. Järvinen M. Epidemiology of tendon injuries in sports. Clin Sports Med 1992;11(3):493–504.
2. Maffulli N, Kader D. Tendinopathy of tendo achillis. J Bone Joint Surg [Br] 2002;84(1):1–8.
3. Astrom M. Partial rupture in chronic Achilles tendinopathy. A retrospective analysis of 342 cases. Acta Orthop Scand 1998;69(4):404–7.
4. Simmonds FA. The diagnosis of the ruptured Achilles tendon. Practitioner 1957;179:56–8.
5. Matles AL. Rupture of the tendo Achilles. Another diagnostic sign. Bull Hosp Joint Dis 1975;36:48–51.
6. Teitz CC, Garrett WEJ, Miniaci A, et al. Tendon problems in athletic individuals. Instr Course Lectures 1997;46:569–82.
7. Maffulli N, Kenward MG, Testa V, et al. The clinical diagnosis of Achilles tendinopathy. Clin J Sport Med 2003;13:11–15.
8. Binfield PM, Maffulli N. Surgical management of common tendinopathies of the lower limb. Sports Exerc Injury 1997;3:116–22.
9. Schepsis AA, Wagner C, Leach RE. Surgical management of Achilles tendon overuse injuries: a long-term follow-up study. Am J Sports Med 1994;22:611–9.
10. Åström M, Westlin N. No effect of piroxicam on Achilles tendinopathy. A randomized study of 70 patients. Acta Orthop Scand 1992;63:631–4.
11. Gill SS, Gelbke MK, Mattson SL, et al. Fluoroscopically guided low-volume peritendinous corticosteroid injection for Achilles tendinopathy. A safety study. J Bone Joint Surg [Am] 2004;86A:802–6.
12. Alfredson H, Lorentzon R. Chronic Achilles tendinosis. Recommendations for treatment and prevention. Sports Med 2000;29:135–46.
13. Rompe JD, Nafa B, Furia JP, . Eccentric loading, shock-wave treatment, or a wait-and-see policy for tendinopathy of the main body of tendo Achillis: a randomized controlled trial. Am J Sports Med 2007;35(3):374–83.
14. Maffulli N, Sharma P, Luscombe KL. Achilles tendinopathy: aetiology and management. J R Soc Med 2004;97(10):472–6.
15. Paavola M, Kannus P, Paakkala T, et al. Long-term prognosis of patients with Achilles tendinopathy. Am J Sports Med 2001;28(5):634–42.
16. Benazzo F, Maffulli N. An operative approach to Achilles tendinopathy. Sports Med Arthrosc Rev 2000;8:96–101.
17. Nelen G, Burssens A. Surgical treatment of chronic Achilles tendonitis. Am J Sports Med 1989;17:754–9.
18. Friedrich T, Schmidt W, Jungmichel D, et al. Histopathology in rabbit Achilles tendon after operative tenolysis (longitudinal fiber incisions). Scand J Med Sci Sports 2001;11(1):4–8.
19. Anderson DL, Taunton JE, Davidson RG. Surgical management of chronic Achilles tendonitis. Clin J Sport Med 1992;2(1):39–42.
20. Calder JD, Saxby TS. Surgical treatment of insertional Achilles tendinosis. Foot Ankle Int 2003;24(2):119–21.
21. Maffulli N, Testa V, Capasso G, et al. Results of percutaneous longitudinal tenotomy for Achilles tendinopathy in middle- and long-distance runners. Am J Sports Med 1997;25:835–40.
22. Testa V, Capasso G, Benazzo F, et al. Management of Achilles tendinopathy by ultrasound-guided percutaneous tenotomy. Med Sci Sports Exerc 2002;34:573–80.

16

Open Debridement of Noninsertional Achilles Tendinopathy

Mark E. Easley and Ian L.D. Le

Although symptomatic Achilles tendinopathy can be managed nonoperatively,[1,2] histologic analysis of tissue obtained at the time of surgery demonstrates degenerative fibrous tissue, no inflammatory cells, and no healing response.[3,4] Surgical management of noninsertional Achilles tendinopathy is indicated when nonoperative management fails. Surgical options for noninsertional Achilles tendinopathy include the following:

1. Percutaneous tenotomy
2. Tenosynovectomy
3. Open Achilles debridement with repair of the residual Achilles tendon
4. Open Achilles debridement with reconstruction of the residual Achilles tendon

Percutaneous tenotomy can be applied to any case of Achilles tendinopathy, but is perhaps best reserved for mild-to-moderate Achilles tendinopathy.[5–7] Open debridement affords a comprehensive evaluation and debridement of the diseased Achilles tendon, with the option for augmentation of the repair or reconstruction, and includes tenosynovectomy in virtually all cases. Following debridement, Achilles tendon repair is generally recommended when 50% or more of the cross-sectional volume of the diseased tendon segment comprises healthy tendon fibers. In contrast, reconstruction or augmentation is typically warranted when the majority of the segment in question is diseased. In approximately 19% to 23% of the cases, a partial rupture of the Achilles tendon will be identified at the segment of tendon in question.[3,8] In a majority of cases, the partial rupture is associated with degenerated/unhealthy tissue. Repair of the partial rupture should be performed in conjunction with excision of the degenerated portion of tendon.

Preoperative Evaluation

The patient generally reports pain in the posterior calf. There is a fusiform thickening within the Achilles tendon substance, located proximal to the Achilles' calcaneal insertion, and the nodule usually limits activities that require push-off during gait. On clinical exam, this tender fusiform mass

J.A. Nunley (ed.), *The Achilles Tendon: Treatment and Rehabilitation*,
DOI: 10.1007/978-1-387-79206-4_16, © Springer Science+Business Media, LLC 2009

is located approximately 4 to 6 cm proximal to the Achilles insertion—the site that is also commonly associated with an acute Achilles tendon rupture. The tendon is noted to be in continuity, and the patient has a negative Thompson test. The painful-arc sign may distinguish between paratendonitis and Achilles tendinopathy.[9] The sign occurs with ankle range of motion, where the tender mass remains localized in paratenonitis, but moves up and down with the Achilles tendon in tendinopathy. While not always present, hyperdorsiflexion of the ankle may be observed in patients with nodular Achilles tendinopathy. Radiographs are of little value, but may reveal calcification within the diseased portion of the tendon. Magnetic resonance imaging (MRI) is not a prerequisite to surgical intervention, but does offer guidance as to the presence and extent of disease, with potentially some prognostic value and reasonable clinical correlation.[10–13]

Isolated paratendonitis[3,14] is not associated with intrasubstance tendon signal change viewed via MRI. However, noninsertional Achilles tendon disorders may exist on a continuum, and therefore pantendonitis may be present, with fluid in the paratenon (paratenonitis) and intrasubstance tendon signal change (tendinopathy) occurring simultaneously. The axial MRI view suggests the extent of tendon disease in the cross section, and the sagittal view demonstrates the extent of tendon disease over the course of the tendon. Likewise, ultrasound has proven effective in determining the extent of tendon disease and may provide some prognostic value and reasonable clinical correlation.[10,15,16] Both MRI and ultrasound may identify a partial rupture at the site of tendon degeneration.[10,15] More recently, MRI has proven effective in monitoring the response to both nonoperative and operative treatments of Achilles tendinopathy.[13,17]

Longitudinal Percutaneous Tenotomy

Background

While not an open technique, percutaneous longitudinal tenotomy bears mentioning in the operative management of noninsertional Achilles tendinopathy. Like nitroglycerine and extracorporeal shockwave therapy, percutaneous tenotomy induces low-grade trauma to the degenerated portion of tendon to stimulate a healing response.[5–7] As it is a minimally invasive technique, percutaneous longitudinal tenotomy may be combined with a brisement[14] (see Chapter 13) to address stenosing tenosynovitis and tendinopathy. Intraoperative ultrasound is applied by some surgeons to identify the exact location of tendon disease when performing percutaneous tenotomy.[6] The minimally invasive nature of this procedure may reduce soft tissue complications associated with open debridement.

Surgical Technique 5–7

Proponents of percutaneous longitudinal tenotomy recommend prone positioning, with the patient's feet protruding beyond the operating table and the ankles supported by a bump (Fig. 16.1A,B). Tourniquet use is unnecessary, and only local anesthesia is required. Via palpation or ultrasound guidance, the diseased tendon segment is identified. In the configuration of the number 5 on a game die, five separate stab incisions are performed in sequence into the

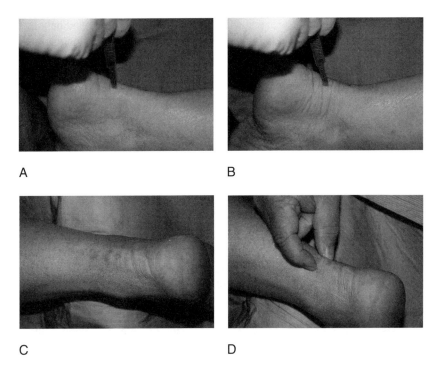

A   B

C   D

Fig. 16.1.A,B Percutaneous longitudinal tenotomies performed into thickened, fusiform portion of Achilles tendon. (A) Scalpel inserted percutaneously through the Achilles, directed proximally, and ankle is dorsiflexed. (B) Same position with ankle plantarflexed. This procedure is repeated in the same location with the scalpel redirected distally and the dorsiflexion/plantarflexion repeated. Then, the technique is repeated in four more locations within the thickened, fusiform portion of the tendon. (C) Appearance of the tendon 8 months following percutaneous longitudinal tenotomy. (D) Some residual thickening is evident, but the tenderness is resolved

diseased tendon using a size 11 surgical scalpel blade. With each introduction of the knife, the blade is held stationary while the ankle is passively dorsiflexed and plantarflexed; and for each incision, the knife blade is introduced twice—the first time with the blade facing distally and the second with the blade directed proximally. The stab incisions are spaced approximately 2 cm from one another. Alternatively, with ultrasound guidance, a single, central stab incision can serve to create multiple tenotomies by angling the blade with each introduction. [6] The wounds are covered with Steri-Strips, and a mildly compressive dressing and a protective bandage are applied (Fig. 16.1C,D).

Open Achilles Tendon Debridement with Repair

Positioning/Tourniquet Use/Anesthesia

The patient may be positioned either prone or supine with a bump under the opposite hip. A tourniquet is optional. If a tourniquet is utilized, a thigh tourniquet offers the advantage over a calf tourniquet of preserving unrestricted gastrocnemius-soleus mobility during surgery. Anesthesia ranges from regional to general and is dictated by surgeon preference and tourniquet use. We prefer to place the patient in the prone position, use a thigh tourniquet, and have the anesthesiologist administer a lumbar plexus/sciatic/femoral regional block. Typically, we exsanguinate the operative extremity with the patient supine on the stretcher, and inflate the tourniquet prior to prepping/draping and positioning the patient in the prone position. While this sequence consumes a few extra minutes of tourniquet time, it is safer for the patient's lumbar spine that otherwise would need to be hyperextended to exsanguinate the extremity.

Surgical Approach

A longitudinal incision is made immediately posteromedial to the diseased portion of the Achilles tendon, extending approximately 2 cm proximal and distal to the fusiform tendon mass (Fig. 16.2). Careful soft tissue handling is important, as the blood supply to the skin in this area is not robust. At no point is forceful traction applied to the skin edges, and forceps are only used on tissues deep to the epidermis. Delamination of the dermal layer from the paratenon overlying the Achilles tendon is minimized. The paratenon is exposed and longitudinally divided directly over the fusiform mass within the tendon (Fig. 16.3). With long-standing paratenonitis, the paratenon may be adherent to the underlying tendon; separation of the paratenon and tendon usually is still possible, but may be difficult. Several small-diameter tagging sutures may be placed in the paratenon to facilitate closure of the paratenon at the completion of the surgery (Fig. 16.4). The following adjacent structures are at risk and must be protected: the sural nerve, the tibial nerve, and the posterior tibial artery. We do not recommend routinely identifying these structures as it requires greater dissection, but the surgeon must maintain an awareness of the close proximity of these structures at risk.

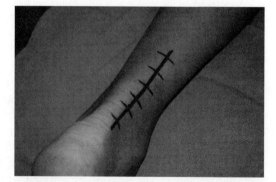

Fig. 16.2. Medial longitudinal approach adjacent to the fusiform thickening of the Achilles tendon

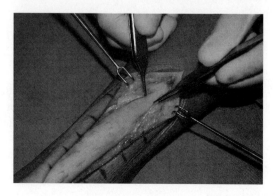

Fig. 16.3. Exposure and reflection of the paratenon

Fig. 16.4. Identifying (and protecting) the sural nerve

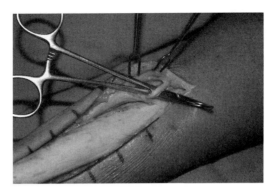

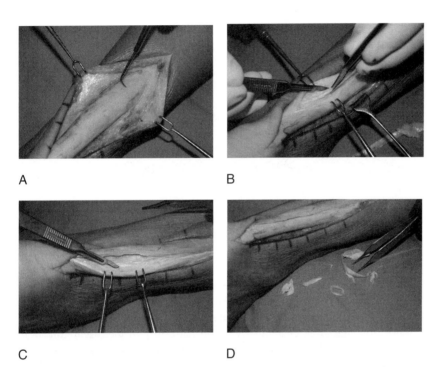

A   B

C   D

Fig. 16.5. (A) Longitudinal incision directly into the focus of the Achilles tendinopathy. (B) Debridement of the diseased portion of the tendon, leaving only healthy Achilles tendon fibers. Note that diseased fibers are typically centrally located. (C) Repair of the remaining healthy Achilles tendon. (D) "Hollow" Achilles tendon. "Tubularized" tendon

Achilles Tendon Debridement and Repair

The Achilles tendon is incised longitudinally over the segment of tendon in question to expose the diseased tissue. The unhealthy tendon is generally easily distinguished from the healthy tendon fibers (Fig. 16.5). Unhealthy, degenerated tissue has a "crabmeat" appearance without distinct orientation in contrast to the healthy, longitudinally organized, collagen fibers of a normal tendon. Although the temptation is great to avoid excessive debridement to preserve adequate tendon substance, leaving diseased tendon most likely results in persistent symptoms. All of the unhealthy fibers must be removed, even if augmentation is thereby necessitated. Often the unhealthy tissue is enucleated, leaving a rim of healthy fibers at the diseased segment (Fig. 16.6).

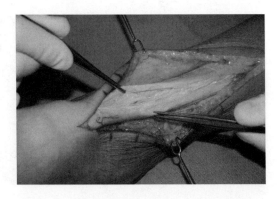

Fig. 16.6. Repair with nonabsorbable suture. Note reestablishment of near-physiologic dimension of Achilles tendon

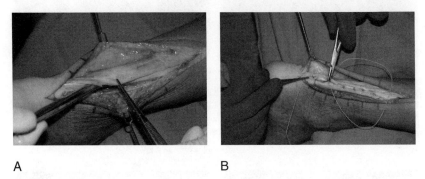

A   B

Fig. 16.7. (A) Repair of the paratenon. Proximal reapproximation of the paratenon. (B) Sural nerve identified and protected. Distal reapproximation of the paratenon

Should a partial tear of the Achilles tendon be identified, repair is indicated, but only after the degenerated/unhealthy tissue is fully debrided.

Repair of the residual healthy Achilles tendon without augmentation is an intraoperative decision. Generally, when at least 50% of the diseased tendon segment is occupied by healthy fibers, a repair is recommended. We perform a common tendon repair technique known as "tubularization" (Fig. 16.7). The healthy tendon fibers are imbricated to create a tubular appearance to the tendon, thereby reinforcing and contouring the tendon at the site of previous pathology. Nonabsorbable suture is recommended, and attempts may be made to bury the knots of these tendons within the imbrication. However, burying these knots is not always possible.

Achilles Tendon Debridement and Reconstruction

Should less than 50% healthy tendon remain following debridement of the diseased segment, reconstruction/augmentation must be considered. We prefer to augment the repair with a flexor hallucis longus (FHL) tendon, a technique introduced by Wapner et al.[18] for management of chronic Achilles tendon ruptures. The FHL tendon is in close proximity and represents the second strongest flexor of the ankle. Harvest of the FHL requires a deep compartment fasciotomy, directly anterior to the Achilles tendon. The FHL muscle is visible through the deep fascia, and the longitudinal fasciotomy can be safely performed directly over this muscle. The posteromedial neurovascular bundle lies directly medial to the FHL tendon, and must be protected.

With the tibial nerve and posterior tibial artery identified and protected, the FHL is harvested. Surgeon preference dictates whether a short or long FHL harvest is performed. A long harvest requires a separate plantar foot incision, places the medial plantar nerve at risk, and offers approximately 3½ cm more tendon than a short harvest. A long harvest may prove beneficial if the majority of the diseased Achilles tendon segment has to be removed due to extensive disease, thereby potentially affording two strands of augmentation to the defect site. Based on a cadaveric study, a long FHL harvest affords approximately 8 cm of FHL tendon versus 5 cm for a short FHL harvest.[19] Alternatively or additionally, a V-Y advancement or turndown procedure, as described for chronic, neglected Achilles tendon ruptures, may be employed (see Chapters 10 and 12).

With a short FHL harvest, the ankle and toes are maximally plantarflexed, the posteromedial neurovascular bundle is protected, and the FHL is transected as far distally as possible within its fibro-osseous tunnel in the posteromedial ankle/foot. The FHL tendon is then secured distally, either directly to the distal Achilles tendon, or anchored to the calcaneus, just anterior to the distal Achilles tendon. We prefer to anchor the FHL to the calcaneus using a bioabsorbable interference screw technique. With the posteromedial neurovascular bundle protected, a tunnel is created in the calcaneus from dorsal to plantar with increasingly larger diameter drill bits/reamers. Proper position for the tunnel is determined on intraoperative fluoroscopy with the initial small diameter drill bit. Final tunnel diameter is dictated by the size of the FHL tendon and the desired interference screw. A nonabsorbable suture is placed in the end of the FHL tendon and passed through the tunnel to the plantar heel using a long needle. With the desired tension (usually with the ankle slightly plantarflexed), the interference screw is placed in the calcaneal tunnel. Several additional nonabsorbable sutures are passed side to side from the FHL tendon to the distal Achilles tendon and to the surrounding calcaneal periosteum. The suture protruding from the heel is tensioned, cut flush with the skin, and allowed to retract.

A long FHL harvest allows for the tendon augmentation to be passed through a calcaneal tunnel so that two portions of the FHL tendon can be used to augment the previous site of tendon disease. This FHL tendon can then be sewn side-to-side to the residual Achilles tendon and to itself; alternatively, it can be woven through the residual Achilles tendon.

Closure

After irrigation, the paratenon is closed over the repair, usually with a running locked absorbable suture (Fig. 16.8). The previously placed tag sutures facilitate identification of the paratenon and its proper alignment during closure. The tourniquet should be released prior to wound closure to ensure meticulous hemostasis and avoid hematoma formation that may induce wound complications. With careful soft tissue handling, the subcutaneous layer is closed, avoiding excessive skin traction or trapping the sural nerve. The skin can be reapproximated with a monofilament suture or staples. Use of a drain is according to the surgeon's preference. Sterile dressings, adequate padding, and a posterior splint are applied with the patient's ankle at the resting tension.

Fig. 16.8. Repair reinforced with absorbable suture

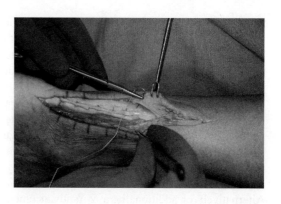

Aftercare

The postoperative course is dictated by (1) wound healing, (2) strength of the repair/reconstruction, and (3) patient compliance. Ideally, range-of-motion should be initiated as early as possible, but it should not compromise skin healing and the repair/fixation.

Percutaneous Tenotomy[5,7]

Postoperative day 1: elevation, nonsteroidal antiinflammatory drugs (NSAIDs), protected weight bearing (WB), isometric strength training with active dorsiflexion and plantarflexion

Postoperative day 2: weight bearing as tolerated (WBAT) with crutches, continue isometric strength training

Week 1: full weight bearing (FWB), continue isometric strength training

Week 2: swimming, water running

Week 4: stationary bike, gentle running; isometric, concentric, eccentric calf muscle strengthening

Weeks 10 to 12: unrestricted return to sports

Open Debridement and Repair

Weeks 1 and 2: elevation, non–weight-bearing (NWB) splinting in slight plantar-flexion (resting tension)

Weeks 3 and 4: if wound healed, touch-down weight bearing (TDWB) gentle range-of-motion exercises without resistance

Weeks 5 and 6: TDWB, isometric, concentric, eccentric calf muscle strengthening

Weeks 7 to 12: progressive WB, stationary bike, water running, continue calf strengthening

Weeks 13 to 16: gentle running, increase resistance exercises

Weeks 17 to 20: unrestricted return to sports

Open Debridement and Reconstruction

The following schedule must be tempered by the quality of the reconstruction/fixation of augmentation:

Weeks 1 and 2: elevation, NWB splinting in slight plantarflexion (resting tension)

Weeks 3 to 6: if wound healed, TDWB gentle range-of-motion exercises without resistance

Weeks 7 to 12: gradual progression of partial weight bearing to FWB, stationary
bike, water running; isometric, concentric, eccentric calf muscle strengthening
Weeks 13 to 20: FWB, gentle running, increase resistance exercises
Weeks 21 to 24: unrestricted return to sports

Complications

Wound Complications

Drawing from the literature reporting open management of Achilles tendon
disorders, including acute Achilles tendon repair, the wound complication rate
is approximately 10%. Wound complications include wound edge necrosis,
hematoma formation, associated superficial wound infections, and symptomatic fibrosis/scar formation. In the majority of cases, these wound complications can be effectively managed with local wound care, wound healing
agents, and extending the period of immobilization. When there is no response
to local wound care, plastic surgery consultation is indicated. There should be little delay in plastic surgery consultation, since physiologically there is very
little soft tissue coverage over the repaired/reconstructed Achilles tendon.
If the paratenon was effectively reapproximated, a wound VAC can prove
effective in avoiding tissue transfer procedures.

Infection

The reported prevalence of superficial wound infections following open
Achilles tendon surgery ranges from less than 1% to almost 20%; for deep
wound infections, the prevalence has been reported to be 2.2%.[20–23] These
estimates combine reports of surgical management of Achilles tendon disorders,
including acute rupture, neglected ruptures, and tendinopathy. Superficial
wound infections can often be managed with topical antibiotic ointments
and oral antibiotics. As for wound complications, if in close follow-up the
response to local wound care is ineffective, the threshold for surgical management should be low. Irrigation and debridement followed by local wound care
or wound VAC management may prove effective for infections not violating
the paratenon.

Deep infections necessitate takedown of the repair/reconstruction and removal
of nonabsorbable sutures. Although unfortunate, removal of all foreign bodies is
essential. Within the paratenon, an inadequately treated infection could readily
spread to infect the entire gastrocnemius/soleus complex.

Rupture

As previously noted, occasionally the degenerated portion of Achilles tendon
develops a partial rupture. In fact, there is histologic evidence that suggests
that degenerated tendons are predisposed to rupture. Therefore, it is essential
to excise all of the degenerated tendon at the index procedure, even if that
necessitates creating an intercalary defect within the tendon. Martin et al.[24]
completely excised the involved segment of tendon in all cases, and bridged
the defect with a long FHL transfer (double-strand) without reestablishing
continuity of the two ends of the Achilles tendon. Although their conclusions
rely on follow-up by questionnaire in some of their patients, the authors report

no cases of reconstruction FHL rupture. Their finding of no FHL ruptures is supported by Wilcox et al.[25]

Persistent Pain

Reported persistent pain following these procedures ranges from 0% to 15%. Not all Achilles tendinopathy is symptomatic, so the exact cause of pain prior to the index procedure is perhaps not fully understood. However, it is generally accepted that symptoms are secondary to the patient having to rely on unhealthy, degenerated tissue over a segment of Achilles tendon during push-off. Accordingly, persistent pain is generally attributed to incomplete resection of diseased tendon. To ensure satisfactory removal of diseased tendon, some surgeons routinely create an intercalary defect in the area of tendon degeneration and then bridge the defect with Achilles tendon advancement or tendon transfer.[24]

Occasionally, sural neuralgia is experienced postoperatively. Since most surgeons use a medial approach to the diseased portion of tendon and elevate the paratenon, direct injury to the sural nerve is relatively uncommon. More likely, scar formation postoperatively results in an adhesive neuralgia. While direct trauma to the sural nerve can be diagnosed clinically within the first few weeks after surgery, adhesive neuralgia may not become apparent for several months. Proper soft tissue handling with deep retraction may lead to a traction neuralgia of the sural nerve, a phenomenon that typically resolves over several weeks to months postoperatively.

Loss of Toe Push-off Strength (Following Flexor Hallucis Longus Transfer)

Transfer of the FHL tendon to augment/reconstruct the Achilles tendon should result in loss of great toe push-off strength. Coull et al.[26] studied the effects of FHL transfer for Achilles tendinopathy and chronic Achilles tendon ruptures in 16 patients. Despite pedobarographic evaluation suggesting a trend toward a reduction in peak pressure loading on the distal phalanx, AOFAS hallux metatarsophalangeal-interphalangeal (MTP-IP) scores and Short Form (SF)-36 questionnaire data failed to demonstrate functional deficits of the hallux in this limited group of patients.

Results

Overview

Reported results of operative management of nodular Achilles tendinopathy are supported almost exclusively by no more than level IV evidence (case series) and are frequently clouded by the fact that several studies include results for treatment of both insertional and noninsertional Achilles tendinopathy. However, our review of the following studies provides some indication of anticipated results in the surgical management of noninsertional Achilles tendinopathy.

Meta-Analysis

In an analysis of 26 studies that report the results of surgical management of Achilles tendinopathy, Tallon et al.[27] identified a negative correlation between success rate and overall method scores. To reach this conclusion, the authors created a highly reproducible methodology score. Important is their observation that although study methods continue to improve, evidence-based guidelines for this area of research are required to provide accurate outcomes data for the surgical management of Achilles tendinopathy.

Comparative Analysis

In a case-controlled study, Maffulli et al.[28] suggested that athletic patients respond better to operative management than nonathletic patients. In their investigation, 80% of athletes and 52% of nonathletes had good to excellent results, respectively. The nonathletic population had a higher complication rate and 19% of the nonathletic population required reoperations.

Benazzo et al.[29] noted that younger age and a relatively short duration of Achilles tendon symptoms was associated with a more favorable outcome with operative intervention in the management of Achilles tendinopathy. The authors concluded that shorter duration of symptoms correlated with less Achilles tendon pathology.

Open Debridement and Repair

Maffulli et al.[30] reported results in 14 athletes undergoing surgical excision of central core degenerative lesions after failing an exhaustive regimen of nonoperative measures. At a mean follow-up of 35 months, only five patients had an excellent or good result. Even reoperation in six patients failed to improve the outcome. Based on this limited patient population, the authors suggested that longstanding disease—an average of 87 months from onset of symptoms to surgical management in this cohort—may have a negative impact on outcome. In fact, they extrapolated to recommend that perhaps earlier surgical intervention should be indicated.

Johnston et al.[14] reported the management of 41 patients with Achilles tendinopathy and an average duration of symptoms of 14 weeks. Approximately 50% responded to nonsurgical management over an 18-week period, and an additional three patients recovered satisfactory function following a brisement procedure. The remaining 17 patients failing nonoperative management underwent tenosynovectomy and limited tendon debridement for tendinosis; all patients managed surgically returned to full function at an average of 31 weeks. Patients responding to nonoperative management tended to be younger (average age 33 years) than those managed surgically (average age 48 years).

Ohberg et al.[31] studied recovery of calf muscle strength following surgically managed noninsertional Achilles tendinopathy in 24 patients. Using concentric and eccentric peak torque measures, the authors noted that calf strength deficits in the affected extremity, compared to the uninvolved extremity observed preoperatively, persisted at an average follow-up of 5 years, despite a rigorous calf-strengthening rehabilitation protocol. The authors concluded that the deficits may be clinically insignificant, since 92% of the patients reported no functional deficits at final follow-up.

Leach et al.[32] noted successful long-term outcomes in nine competitive runners undergoing surgical debridement and repair for noninsertional Achilles tendinopathy. Although all patients returned to their desired high level of function, two required reoperation to achieve that status.

Saxena and Cheung[33,34] reported that athletic patients, particularly male runners, tended to return to their desired level of activity more rapidly than nonathletic patients. Two retrospective reviews comprised a variety of diagnoses accounting for achillodynia, including noninsertional tendinopathy, insertional tendinopathy, and tenosynovitis. Patients undergoing surgical management requiring bony procedures (insertional) necessitated the greatest time to return to full activity (average 18.6 weeks). Patients with noninsertional Achilles tendinopathy (undergoing excision/repair procedures) returned to full activity by an average of 13.2 weeks for mucoid degeneration and 14.4 weeks for calcific tendinosis. Reconstructive procedures for chronic Achilles tendon ruptures returned at an average of 34.0 weeks. In contrast, patients without tendinopathy and only paratenonitis, undergoing tenolysis/tenosynovectomy only, returned to desired level of function on average by 7.7 weeks.

Schepsis et al.[35] reviewed a wide variety of Achilles tendon pathology managed surgically, and noted that surgical management of tendinopathy yielded the lowest percentage of satisfactory outcomes. The cohort of 79 patients comprised a relatively active patient population, average age 33 years (range, 17 to 59 years), with diagnoses of paratenonitis ($n = 23$), noninsertional tendinopathy ($n = 15$), retrocalcaneal bursitis ($n = 24$), insertional tendinopathy ($n = 7$), and combined findings ($n = 10$). Good to excellent outcomes were as follows: paratenonitis (87%), insertional tendinopathy (8%), retrocalcaneal bursitis (75%), and noninsertional tendinopathy (67%). Furthermore, the noninsertional tendinopathy group also required the highest number of reoperations.

In a prospective study, Paavola et al.[36] demonstrated a more favorable outcome for surgical management of peritendinous adhesions than peritendinous adhesions associated with tendinopathy. At relatively short-term follow-up (7 months), of the 42 patients evaluated preoperatively and at 7 months or later, satisfactory results were 88% for the group with peritendinous adhesions and 54% for the groups with peritendinous adhesions and tendinosis. Likewise, the incidence of complications was 6% for the peritendinous adhesion group and 27% for the group with peritendinous adhesions and tendinosis.

In two separate studies, Alfredson et al.[37,38] prospectively demonstrated, following surgical management of Achilles tendinopathy, that for the recovery of plantarflexion muscle strength to equal that of the unaffected side takes in excess of 6 months and may require 1 year. Evaluation focused on concentric and eccentric peak torque measures. The investigators could not identify any differences in outcome if the surgically managed tendon was immobilized for 2 weeks or 6 weeks in the immediate postoperative period.

Surgical management of isolated tenosynovitis, or tenosynovitis without associated tendinopathy, almost uniformly yields a favorable outcome with a relatively rapid return to desired functional level. Gould and Korson[39] reported successful outcomes with return to full function within only a few months in eight of nine patients undergoing excision of a pseudosheath of degenerative tissue that was creating a stenosing tenosynovitis.

Results of reconstruction using an FHL augmentation for inadequate residual healthy tendons have been favorable.[24,25] At an average followup of 14 months, Wilcox et al.[25] reported that 90% of their 20 patients undergoing debridement and FHL augmentation for noninsertional Achilles tendinopathy scored 70 points or higher on the AOFAS hindfoot-ankle score. No wound complications, ruptures, or recurrences of tendinopathy were reported. Although the

SF-36 outcomes measure for physical function was lower than that for United States norms, the authors suggested FHL reconstruction is a reasonable option for reconstruction of Achilles tendinopathy.

Martin et al.[24] reported the results of 56 surgically managed Achilles tendinopathies in 44 patients. In all cases, complete excision of the diseased portion of tendon was performed, and the defect was spanned via an FHL tendon transfer. Although over half of the patients responded only by questionnaire and only 19 were examined at final follow-up, the authors concluded that the SF-36 scores of their surgically managed patients were not statistically significantly different from scores for the general United States population. This conclusion was made even though plantarflexion range of motion and plantarflexion strength were significantly less than the unaffected side in the 19 patients tested. In these 19 patients, the average AOFAS score was 91 points. Pain was decreased in 96% ($n = 42$) and satisfaction was 86% ($n = 38$).

Percutaneous Longitudinal Tenotomy

In three separate investigations of athletic patients with Achilles tendinopathy with an average follow-up ranging from 16 to 36 months, Testa and Maffulli and coauthors[5–7] reported satisfactory results of percutaneous longitudinal tenotomy, with or without ultrasound guidance, in a majority of patients. Maffulli et al.[5] noted good to excellent results in 77% of middle- to long-distance runners, and Testa et al.[7] observed good to excellent results in 86% of track-and-field athletes. In a separate study, 75% of athletes evaluated after ultrasound-guided percutaneous tenotomy returned to preinjury levels of activity.[6] These authors conclude that percutaneous tenotomy is a reasonably safe outpatient procedure for noninsertional Achilles tendinopathy when nonoperative measures fail. They caution that diffuse or multinodular tendinopathy or pantendinopathy may be better managed with open paratenon stripping and multiple longitudinal tenotomies.

References

1. Ohberg L, Alfredson H. Effects on neovascularisation behind the good results with eccentric training in chronic mid-portion Achilles tendinosis? Knee Surg Sports Traumatol Arthrosc 2004;12(5):465–70.
2. Ohberg L, Lorentzon R, Alfredson H. Eccentric training in patients with chronic Achilles tendinosis: normalised tendon structure and decreased thickness at follow up. Br J Sports Med 2004;38(1):8–11.
3. Astrom M, Rausing A. Chronic Achilles tendinopathy. A survey of surgical and histopathologic findings. Clin Orthop Rel Res 1995;(316):151–64.
4. Maffulli N, Kader D. Tendinopathy of tendo achillis. J Bone Joint Surg [Br] 2002;84(1):1–8.
5. Maffulli N, Testa V, Capasso G, et al. Results of percutaneous longitudinal tenotomy for Achilles tendinopathy in middle- and long-distance runners. Am J Sports Med 1997;25(6):835–40.
6. Testa V, Capasso G, et alBenazzo F, et al. Management of Achilles tendinopathy by ultrasound-guided percutaneous tenotomy. Med Sci Sports Exerc 2002;34(4):573–80.
7. Testa V, Maffulli N, Capasso G, et al. Percutaneous longitudinal tenotomy in chronic Achilles tendonitis. Bull Hosp Joint Dis 1996;54(4):241–4.
8. Astrom M. Partial rupture in chronic Achilles tendinopathy. A retrospective analysis of 342 cases. Acta Orthop Scand 1998;69(4):404–7.

9. Maffulli N, Wong J, Almekinders LC. Types and epidemiology of tendinopathy. Clin Sports Med 2003;22(4):675–92.
10. Astrom M, Gentz CF, Nilsson P, et al. Imaging in chronic Achilles tendinopathy: a comparison of ultrasonography, magnetic resonance imaging and surgical findings in 27 histologically verified cases. Skeletal Radiol 1996;25(7):615–20.
11. Karjalainen PT, Soila K, Aronen HJ, et al. MR imaging of overuse injuries of the Achilles tendon. AJR Am J Roentgenol 2000;175(1):251–60.
12. Gardin A, Bruno J, Movin T, et al. Magnetic resonance signal, rather than tendon volume, correlates to pain and functional impairment in chronic Achilles tendinopathy. Acta Radiol 2006;47(7):718–24.
13. Shalabi A, Kristoffersen-Wilberg M, Svensson L, et al. Eccentric training of the gastrocnemius-soleus complex in chronic Achilles tendinopathy results in decreased tendon volume and intratendinous signal as evaluated by MRI. Am J Sports Med 2004;32(5):1286–96.
14. Johnston E, Scranton P Jr, Pfeffer GB. Chronic disorders of the Achilles tendon: results of conservative and surgical treatments. Foot Ankle Int 1997;18(9):570–4.
15. Lehtinen A, Peltokallio P, et alTaavitsainen M. Sonography of Achilles tendon correlated to operative findings. Ann Chir Gynaecol 1994;83(4):322–7.
16. Paavola M, Paakkala T, Kannus P, et al. Ultrasonography in the differential diagnosis of Achilles tendon injuries and related disorders. A comparison between pre-operative ultrasonography and surgical findings. Acta Radiol 1998;39(6):612–9.
17. Shalabi A, Kristoffersen-Wiberg M, Papadogiannakis N, et al. Dynamic contrast-enhanced MR imaging and histopathology in chronic Achilles tendinosis. A longitudinal MR study of 15 patients. Acta Radiol 2002;43(2):198–206.
18. Wapner KL, Pavlock GS, Hecht PJ, et al. Repair of chronic Achilles tendon rupture with flexor hallucis longus tendon transfer. Foot Ankle 1993;14(8):443–9.
19. Tashjian RZ, Hur J, Sullivan RJ, et al. Flexor hallucis longus transfer for repair of chronic Achilles tendinopathy. Foot Ankle Int 2003;24(9):673–6.
20. Khan RJ, Fick D, Keogh A, et al. Treatment of acute Achilles tendon ruptures. A meta-analysis of randomized, controlled trials. J Bone Joint Surg [Am] 2005;87(10):2202–10.
21. Paavola M, Orava S, Leppilahti J, et al. Chronic Achilles tendon overuse injury: complications after surgical treatment. An analysis of 432 consecutive patients. Am J Sports Med 2000;28(1):77–82.
22. Pajala A, Kangas J, Ohtonen P, et al. Rerupture and deep infection following treatment of total Achilles tendon rupture. J Bone Joint Surg [Am] 2002;84-A(11):2016–21.
23. Chiodo CP, Wilson MG. Current concepts review: acute ruptures of the Achilles tendon. Foot Ankle Int 2006;27(4):305–13.
24. Martin RL, Manning CM, Carcia CR, et al. An outcome study of chronic Achilles tendinosis after excision of the Achilles tendon and flexor hallucis longus tendon transfer. Foot Ankle Int 2005;26(9):691–7.
25. Wilcox DK, Bohay DR, Anderson JG. Treatment of chronic Achilles tendon disorders with flexor hallucis longus tendon transfer/augmentation. Foot Ankle Int 2000;21(12):1004–10.
26. Coull R, Flavin R, Stephens MM. Flexor hallucis longus tendon transfer: evaluation of postoperative morbidity. Foot Ankle Int 2003;24(12):931–4.
27. Tallon C, Coleman BD, Khan KM, et al. Outcome of surgery for chronic Achilles tendinopathy. A critical review. Am J Sports Med 2001;29(3):315–20.
28. Maffulli N, Testa V, Capasso G, et al. Surgery for chronic Achilles tendinopathy yields worse results in nonathletic patients. Clin J Sport Med 2006;16(2):123–8.
29. Benazzo F, Stennardo G, Valli M. Achilles and patellar tendinopathies in athletes: pathogenesis and surgical treatment. Bull Hosp Joint Dis 1996;54(4):236–40.
30. Maffulli N, Binfield PM, Moore D, et al. Surgical decompression of chronic central core lesions of the Achilles tendon. Am J Sports Med 1999;27(6):747–52.

31. Ohberg L, Lorentzon R, Alfredson H. Good clinical results but persisting side-to-side differences in calf muscle strength after surgical treatment of chronic Achilles tendinosis: a 5-year follow-up. Scand J Med Sci Sports 2001;11(4):207–12.
32. Leach RE, Schepsis AA, Takai H. Long-term results of surgical management of Achilles tendinitis in runners. Clin Orthop Rel Res 1992;(282):208–12.
33. Saxena A, Cheung S. Surgery for chronic Achilles tendinopathy. Review of 91 procedures over 10 years. J Am Podiatr Med Assoc 2003;93(4):283–91.
34. Saxena A. Results of chronic Achilles tendinopathy surgery on elite and nonelite track athletes. Foot Ankle Int 2003;24(9):712–20.
35. Schepsis AA, Jones H, Haas AL. Achilles tendon disorders in athletes. Am J Sports Med 2002;30(2):287–305.
36. Paavola M, Kannus P, Orava S, et al. Surgical treatment for chronic Achilles tendinopathy: a prospective seven month follow up study. Br J Sports Med 2002;36(3):178–82.
37. Alfredson H, Pietila T, Lorentzon R. Chronic Achilles tendinitis and calf muscle strength. Am J Sports Med 199624(6):829–33.
38. Alfredson H, Pietila T, Ohberg L, et al. Achilles tendinosis and calf muscle strength. The effect of short-term immobilization after surgical treatment. Am J Sports Med 1998;26(2):166–71.
39. Gould N, Korson R. Stenosing tenosynovitis of the pseudosheath of the tendo Achilles. Foot Ankle Int 2002;23(7):595–9.

17

Overview of Insertional Achilles Tendinopathy

James A. Nunley

Overuse injury of the Achilles tendon is becoming a more common problem in the United States as the younger population becomes more athletic and as elderly patients assume ever-increasing levels of physical activity. Thus, it is not surprising that the Achilles tendon, one of the largest tendons in the body, would be subjected to repetitive overuse injuries in both patient populations. This overuse phenomenon can ultimately lead to different forms of Achilles tendinopathy. It is important at the onset to emphasize that Achilles tendinopathy is not a single entity, but rather is made up of a large variety of pathophysiologic processes, all of which can result in pain production at the posterior heel and calf areas. It is useful, I believe, to divide Achilles tendinopathy into noninsertional and insertional disease processes since the location of the pain and the pathophysiology is so distinctly different. This chapter concentrates on the evaluation and diagnostic characteristics of insertional Achilles tendinopathy.

The term *insertional Achilles tendinosis* was originally suggested by Clain and Baxter,[1] who felt that this condition was an overuse phenomenon that resulted in enthesopathic changes occurring within the Achilles tendon. The theory was that repetitive mechanical stress from overuse would lead to microtears within the tendon itself. Given the low-oxygen environment seen in that anatomic area of the Achilles tendon, this subsequently would cause localized collagen degeneration, fibrosis, and, ultimately, calcification. Schepsis and Leach[2] also noted that insertional tendinosis is frequently seen in combination with Haglund's deformity and symptomatic retrocalcaneal bursitis, which they believed would exacerbate the condition simply by mechanical bony impingement and chemical irritation. The result in any case is the production of posterior heel pain.

The posterior heel is composed of the Achilles tendon insertion, the posterior superior calcaneal process, and the retrocalcaneal bursa. The Achilles fibers insert at the enthesis on the posterior-inferior aspect of the calcaneus by way of Sharpey's fibers. The insertion of the tendon is quite broad and extends very far distally on the calcaneus. In our study, the distance over which the Achilles inserts measured from superior to inferior is 19.8 mm (range, 13 to 25 mm) and the width measured at the superior insertion is 23.8 mm (range,

J.A. Nunley (ed.), *The Achilles Tendon: Treatment and Rehabilitation*,
DOI: 10.1007/978-1-387-79206-4_17, © Springer Science+Business Media, LLC 2009

17 to 30 mm), while at the inferiormost insertion the distance averages 31.2 mm (range, 25 to 38 mm).[3] The retrocalcaneal bursa is a horseshoe-shaped structure that is approximately 22 mm long, 8 mm wide, and 4 mm deep as established by Frye and colleagues,[4] and its function is to lubricate the anterior surface of the Achilles tendon. The superior calcaneal process makes up the final component of the posterior heel region and is generally the superior border of the retrocalcaneal bursa.

Since the space between the Achilles tendon and the calcaneus is occupied by the retrocalcaneal bursa—and the deep surface of the tendon is part of the bursa and the anterior part of the bursa is the calcaneus—during dorsiflexion of the ankle the Achilles tendon bends near its distal attachment and the bursa flattens as its walls become opposed. This allows the distal part of the Achilles tendon to be pressed against the calcaneus. This complex anatomic region, with an extremely important function, is designed to protect the tendon and the bone from excessive wear. It has been established by DePalma et al.[5] that there are three different fibrocartilaginous surfaces that make up this complex interaction: fibrocartilage on the anterior or deep surface of the tendon, which some have referred to as the sesamoid fibrocartilage; periosteal fibrocartilage covering the superior calcaneal tuberosity; and fibrocartilage of the enthesis where the Achilles tendon inserts into bone. Recent investigations have implicated these fibrocartilaginous cells as a factor in the degenerative phenomenon that occurs with posterior heel pain.[5]

Posterior heel pain can certainly be caused by any disease process that affects any one or all three of these components, such as a prominent superior calcaneal process (Haglund's deformity), which has been associated with the retrocalcaneal bursitis that is frequently seen in long-distance runners.[5] There can be mechanical causes for retrocalcaneal bursitis, such as a varus hindfoot and a cavus foot with the resultant increase in calcaneal pitch.[1,7–9] Some patients simply have a prominent posterior lateral superior tuberosity, which aggravates the heel counter of the shoe and has been referred to as "pump bump."[1,8] This is usually seen in women who wear high-heel shoes. Other causes of posterior heel pain that must be included in the differential diagnosis are inflammatory causes such as rheumatoid arthritis, seronegative spondyloarthropathies, and gout; even pseudogout or chondrocalcinosis has been associated with calcium pyrophosphate dehydrate deposition at the Achilles insertion.[10–12]

Patient Presentation

There are two distinct groups of patients with insertional Achilles tendinopathy. The first group is made up primarily of younger athletic individuals. Insertional Achilles tendinopathy is extremely common in runners, ballet dancers, and in virtually all sports that involve running. In his review of runners, Baxter[1,6] reported that Achilles tendonitis was the most common form of tendonitis seen in runners and had an incidence of 6.5% ranging up to 18%. However, Baxter also reported that the majority (54%) of his runners continued to compete despite pain in the Achilles tendon, while only 16% abandoned the sport.[1,6] In these patients, the etiology of the Achilles tendinopathy is frequently felt to be the result of a contracture of the Achilles tendon itself, hyperpronation of the foot, or training errors.

In patients who are hyperpronators, there is increased stress on the medial aspect of the Achilles tendon that occurs with running and walking. This occurs because hyperpronators maintain their foot posture well past mid-stance in both the running and walking gait; thus, there are ever-increasing loads applied to the medial aspect of the calcaneus.[1] Additionally, most running and jogging shoes are flat as opposed to walking shoes, which have a heel. These flat running shoes, of course, lengthen the Achilles tendon and thus increase stress within the tendon in contrast to a shoe with a heel, which will actually decrease tension within the tendon.

Many young athletes also pursue training regimens that are excessive, especially with hill running, which greatly strains the Achilles tendon. They do not allow the tendon sufficient time to recover from minor strains with training, leading to a more chronic condition of pain at the heel and ultimately contracture of the Achilles tendon.

Examination

Physical examination usually reveals tenderness in the region of the posterior calcaneus at the Achilles tendon insertion. There may be visible swelling with overlying erythema and warmth associated with retrocalcaneal bursitis. Frequently, the gastroc-soleus complex is tight, which is manifested by decreased ankle dorsiflexion when compared to the contralateral extremity. Plain radiographic imaging is important to demonstrate not only the Haglund's deformity, but also any associated intratendinous calcification at the bone tendon interface.[13–15] These radiographs should always been obtained with the patient in the standing position.

Treatment

In the younger athlete with insertional Achilles tendinopathy, nonoperative management is usually satisfactory. The usual treatment is rest, ice to reduce inflammation and pain, and stretching to maintain muscle tendon length. Evaluation and adoption of proper athletic shoe wear and the proper use of orthotics when necessary, combined with appropriate coaching instructions and observation of training regimens, frequently are necessary to alleviate the pain. Something as simple as changing the direction that the athlete routinely uses when running around the track can be successful. When the athlete trains by running in the same direction all the time, the athlete is putting increased stress on the outer leg. This may lead to an insertional Achilles tendinopathy, which can be obviated by just simply changing the training program so that the athlete runs on alternate days around the track in the opposite direction. It is also imperative that adequate stretching and warm-up of the muscle tendon units occur before any strenuous exercise. Shoes that are appropriate, not excessively worn, and have adequate cushioning should be recommended for all running athletes.

The older patient who presents with insertional Achilles tendinopathy differs from the young athlete. The older patient tends to be sedentary, less athletic, overweight, and frequently has multiple medical conditions such as hypertension and diabetes.[16]

Pathophysiology

In the older patient with insertional Achilles tendinopathy, the true pathology is one of tendinosis, which is visible microscopically. The Achilles tendon shows attritional degenerative changes and there frequently are cystic alterations of the bone along the posterior calcaneal tuberosity. The hallmark of this disorder is ossification within the Achilles tendon, best seen on a standing lateral radiograph. This ossification occurs most likely because of vertical microtears within the tendon, which occur in a hypoxemic environment where there is inadequate oxygenation and vascularity for complete tendon healing, thus leading to a proliferation of calcified degenerative tendon. This degenerative process is no different from that seen in other areas of the body (e.g., rotator cuff, tennis elbow).

Attempts to treat the patient with insertional Achilles tendinopathy by nonoperative means in this older population, in my experience, has rarely been successful. Attempts to get the patient to wear shoes in which the counter does not rub against the painful Haglund's deformity or the calcified tendon can be helpful. Judicious use of heel lifts to enable the tendon to rest, followed by a stretching regimen, has been employed with some success. Horseshoe-shaped pads and orthotics to cushion and to prevent pressure in the area of tenderness have limited success. It should be remembered that the presence of ossification within the Achilles tendon does not by itself necessarily produce pain. Many individuals present with asymptomatic radiographic calcification in the Achilles tendon, just as one sees the same radiographic calcification in the subcalcaneal region with the posterior heel spur, which is rarely the cause of plantar heel pain. Sources of the pain should be diligently sought in all patients with insertional Achilles tendinopathy.

The pain is frequently caused by a combination of the various sources that would include an inflamed retrocalcaneal bursa; a large Haglund's deformity (superior calcaneal process), which can push against and produce more pressure on the retrocalcaneal bursa as well as on the Achilles tendon; as well as the microtear and degenerative tendinopathy seen within the tendon itself. The surgical approach, when needed to treat insertional Achilles tendinopathy, must necessarily address all the pathology that is producing the pain. There are many different surgical approaches that have been utilized to treat this disorder, including the use of lateral incisions to expose the lateral calcaneal ridge; medial and lateral incisions to remove ossified tendon; the central tendon splitting approach, which allows debridement of the degenerative tendon, retrocalcaneal bursa, and Haglund's deformity to be defined and addressed specifically; arthroscopic bursectomy with removal of the retrocalcaneal bursa and Haglund's deformity; and, finally, complete detachment of the Achilles tendon from its insertion on the calcaneus with debridement of bone and tendon followed by lengthening of the tendon superiorly and reattachment of the tendon distally to the calcaneus.[1,8,17–19] All of these approaches have been utilized successfully by different authors.

There is a third less common type of individual who presents with posterior heel pain and insertional Achilles tendinopathy. These are patients who have an inflammatory enthesopathy. These may be young men with Reiter's syndrome or there may be patients of any age who have a seronegative spondyloarthropathy. This diagnosis should be suspected in individuals with uncharacteristic clinical presentation or in younger individuals with calcified tendons. The treatment of this painful enthesopathy can frequently be managed nonoperatively with medication specific for the spondyloarthropathy. Gerster et al.[10–12] also noted that pseudogout or chondrocalcinosis can produce deposition of calcium pyrophosphate crystals at the Achilles insertion and can be another source of inflammatory enthesopathy.

Some authors have advocated the use of local cortisone, iontophoresis, and ultrasound to treat insertional Achilles tendinopathy. Other authors have recommended cortisone injection only for retrocalcaneal bursitis. I feel that steroid injection in the posterior heel region should be avoided at all cost because of the potential for rupture of the Achilles tendon.[20] A preferable way to use steroids, if the condition warrants, is with an oral short course given over 5 to 7 days. Lastly, in some patients a cast applied for a short period of time will ensure rest, reduce the inflammation, and can also be tried as a nonoperative management.

When nonoperative management fails, surgical treatment is warranted, as described in the following chapters. Generally, surgical treatment has been extremely successful, and there are numerous different approaches to this condition.

References

1. Clain M, Baxter D. Foot fellows reviewer: Achilles tendonitis. Foot Ankle 1992;13:482–7.
2. Schepsis AA, Leach RE. Surgical management of Achilles tendonitis. Am J Sports Medicine 1987;15:308–15.
3. Kolodziej P, Glisson RR, Nunley JA. Risk of avulsion of the Achilles tendon after partial excision for treatment of insertional tendonitis and Haglund's deformity: a biomechanical study. Foot Ankle Int 1999;7:433–7.
4. Frye C, Rosenberg Z, Shereff MJ. The retrocalcaneal bursa: anatomy and veinography. Foot Ankle 1992;13:203–7.
5. dePalma L, Marinelli M, Meme L, et al. Immunohistochemistry of the enthesis organ of the human Achilles tendon. Foot Ankle Int 2004;6:414–8.
6. Baxter DE, Zingas C. The foot in running. J Am Acad Orthop Surg 1995;3:136–45.
7. Dickinson PH, Coutts MB, Woodward EP, et al. Tendo Achillis bursitis. J Bone Joint Surg 1966;48A:77–81.
8. Jones D, James S. Partial calcaneal ostectomy for retrocalcaneal bursitis. Am J Sports Med 1984;12:72–3.
9. McGarvey WC, Palumbo RC, Baxter D. Insertional Achilles tendinosis: surgical treatment through a central tendon splitting approach. Foot Ankle Int 2002;23:19–25.
10. Gerster JG, Baud CA, Lagier R, et al. Tendon calcifications in chondrocalcinosis. Arthritis Rheum 1977;20:717–21.
11. Gerster JG, Lagier R, Boivin G. Achilles tendinitis associated with chondrocalcinosis. J Rheumatol 1980;7:82–7.
12. Gerster JG, Saudan Y, Fallet GH. Talagie: a review of 30 severe cases. J Rheumatol 1978;5:210–6.
13. Lotke P. Ossification of the Achilles tendon. J Bone Joint Surg 1970;52A:157–60.
14. Pavlov H, Henerghan MA, Hersh A, et al. The Haglund syndrome: initial and differential diagnosis. Radiology 1982;144:83–8.
15. Ruch JA. Haglund's disease. J Am Podiatr Assoc 1974;64:1000–3.
16. Holmes G, Lin J. Etiologic factors associated with symptomatic Achilles tendinopathy. Foot Ankle Int 2006;11:1952–9.

17. Angermann P. Chronic retrocalcaneal bursitis, treated by resection of the calcaneus. Foot Ankle 1990;10:285–7.
18. Leitze Z, Sella EJ, Aversar M. Endoscopic compression of the retrocalcaneal space. J Bone Joint Surg 2003;8:1483–96.
19. Sayana M, Maffuli N. Insertional tendinopathy of the Achilles tendon: debridement and reattachment of the Achilles tendon using bone anchors. Tech Foot Ankle Surg;4:209–13.
20. Kennedy J, Willis B. The effects of local steroid injections on tendons: a biomechanical and microscopic correlative study. Am J Sports Med 1976;4:11–21.

18

Medial and Lateral Approaches to Insertional Achilles Disease

W. Hodges Davis

Insertional Achilles disease offers a number of challenges for the surgeon. One of the areas of debate is the optimal surgical approach to deal with the varied pathology in this anatomic area.[1–4] The choice of approach is guided by the anatomic location of the pathology, the need to access non-Achilles structures, and surgeon preference. This chapter describes the medial and lateral approaches to the insertion, as well as the variants of each, based on the anatomy and pathology.

Anatomy

The normal anatomy of the Achilles insertion is unique primarily as to the area of the insertion and the bony anatomy that juxtaposes the tendon. The gastrocnemius and soleus tendons blend together to form a single tendon in the distal posterior calf. The combined tendon (Achilles) rotates internally, placing the soleus fibers more medial and posterior to those of the gastrocnemius. The broad insertion on the flattened surface of the posterior calcaneus completely covers the middle third of this bone and inserts with a combination of calcified and noncalcified fibrocartilage at the distal insertional ridge.[5,6]

The retrocalcaneal bursa is a horseshoe-shaped structure between the tendon and the bone just proximal to the anatomic insertion, which lubricates this junction.[5] The blood supply of the distal tendon comes from the paratenon and from osseous and periosteal vessels in this area. In injection studies, Lagergren and Lindholm[7] showed an abundance of vascularity in this area of the Achilles. The sensory innervation comes from the medial calcaneal branches of the posterior tibial nerve (medial and central, S1, S2) and the sural nerve (lateral and centrolateral, S1, S2).[6]

The topography of the Achilles at its insertion is important for accurate placement of the incisions we will be describing (Fig. 18.1). The tendon transects the posterior ankle and can be easily palpated because of the tendon's subcutaneous course. The tendon inserts into the calcaneus broadly, and the Achilles insertional ridge of the calcaneus is palpated at the distal insertion of the tendon. The posterior calcaneus can be easily palpated medial, lateral, and posterior. The retrocalcaneal space, which is deep to the Achilles at its insertion,

J.A. Nunley (ed.), *The Achilles Tendon: Treatment and Rehabilitation*,
DOI: 10.1007/978-1-387-79206-4_18, © Springer Science+Business Media, LLC 2009

Fig. 18.1. Topographic anatomy of the distal and posterior Achilles tendon. A, distal insertional ridge of the calcaneus; B, Achilles tendon; C, sural nerve; D, posterior tibial nerve and artery

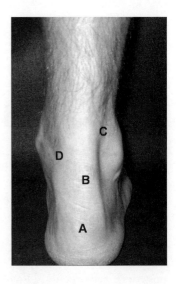

can be easily pinched by pressure from either a medial or lateral direction. The retrocalcaneal space or its bursa is easily delineated from the Achilles proper. The posterior lateral ankle is another access point for the peroneal tendons as they pass posterior to the fibula and can be an easier way to feel both tendons in the fibula groove. The same can be said for the flexor hallucis longus (FHL) tendon, which is a posterior medial ankle tendon at this point.

Pathologic Anatomy

The more salient issue in describing the approach to the distal Achilles is where the pathology is. In calcific Achilles tendonitis, the "spurring" is most often central or centrolateral and rarely medial. For the hypertrophic lateral calcaneal ridge (nicknamed the "pump bump"), the pathology is clearly lateral. The same can be said for recalcitrant retrocalcaneal bursitis.[3,4,8] The medial approach may be favored if there is combined distal Achilles and FHL pathology (or need for FHL transfer).

Lateral Approach

The following are the indications for the lateral approach to the distal Achilles:

1. Lateral calcaneal ridge hypertrophy (pump bump)
2. Retrocalcaneal bursitis
3. Insertional (noncalcific) Achilles tendonitis
4. Calcific Achilles tendonitis
5. Achilles sleeve avulsion type ruptures
6. Distraction arthrodesis of the subtalar joint
7. Posterior Achilles rheumatoid nodules
8. Posterior calcaneal tumors or infections

The anatomic structures at risk for this approach are the following:

1. Sural nerve
2. Lateral Achilles osseous blood supply

Position

The patient position should be prone or lateral.

Technique

The incision for the lateral approach to the insertion of the Achilles is just lateral to the lateral Achilles, proximally, and extends distally to the distal insertional ridge of the calcaneus (Fig. 18.2). The sural nerve can remain millimeters lateral to the Achilles until 4 to 5 cm from the distal insertion. To protect the nerve, the proximal portion of the incision should be carefully explored prior to cutting to bone in order to look for the sural nerve (Fig. 18.3). Most often it will not extend this far distally, but the area should be explored. Once the nerve is either protected or confirmed not to be present, the dissection can be brought sharply to the calcaneus. The periosteum should be sharply dissected from the bone anteriorly (making a periosteal cuff) to allow for good visualization of the contours of the calcaneus (Fig. 18.4). The periosteum can then be dissected posteriorly and laterally, lifting up the lateral edge of the Achilles insertion (Fig. 18.5). If the subperiosteal dissection is made the entire length of the incision, the

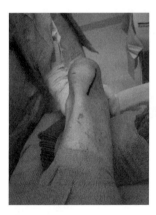
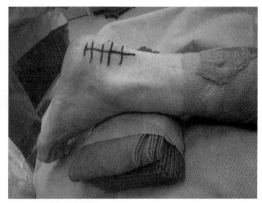

A   B

Fig. 18.2. Placement of incision for lateral approach to the Achilles tendon. (A) Posterior view. (B) Lateral view

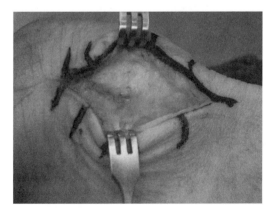

Fig. 18.3. Scissor exploration for possible distal sural nerve extension

Fig. 18.4. Careful dissection of an anterior periosteal sleeve

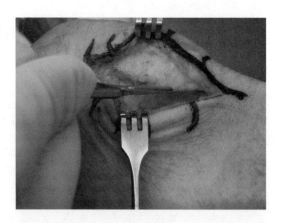

Fig. 18.5. Posterior lateral dissection of Achilles insertion off of the calcaneus

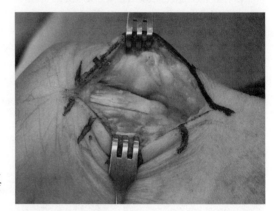

Fig. 18.6. Access to the retrocalcaneal bursa

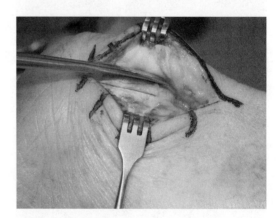

space between the Achilles and the posterior tuberosity of the calcaneus will be exposed. The retrocalcaneal bursa can be accessed at that time (Fig. 18.6).

This approach allows for the dissection between the Achilles and the skin to address pathology in the Achilles bursa (Fig. 18.7). The calcaneus can be addressed safely by lifting up thc Achilles insertion and detaching it up to the center of the posterior calcaneus. This can be done sharply or with a wide elevator, which allows the calcaneus proximal to the insertion to be exposed.

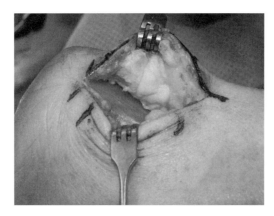

Fig. 18.7. The skin and subcutaneous tissue can be dissected off the distal Achilles to approach the more subcutaneous Achilles

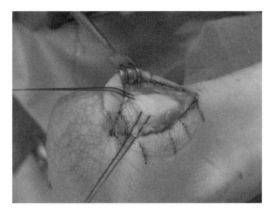

Fig. 18.8. The periosteum is repaired in layers to secure a strong closure

The incision can be safely extended proximally or distally if more of the Achilles or the calcaneus needs to be seen. The closure is done in layers. It is important to repair the periosteal Achilles layer carefully (Fig. 18.8).

The useful variant of the lateral approach requires an extension of the distal incision across to the medial side. This can be done quite distally, and is most often done when distal sleeve rupture repairs require more exposure or when the surgeon did not perceive a need for an FHL transfer preoperatively; this can help with the FHL harvest.

Medial Approach

The following are the indications for the medial approach to the distal Achilles:

1. Achilles pathology requiring an FHL transfer or harvest[2,9]
2. Insertional (noncalcific) Achilles tendonitis
3. Retrocalcaneal bursitis
4. Calcific Achilles tendonitis

5. Achilles sleeve avulsion-type ruptures
6. Posterior Achilles rheumatoid nodules
7. Posterior calcaneal tumors or infections

The anatomic structures at risk for this approach are the following:

1. Medial calcaneal branches of the posterior tibial nerve
2. Medial Achilles osseous blood supply
3. Medial neurovascular bundle
4. Plantaris tendon

Position

The patient position is prone.

Technique

The incision for the medial approach to the Achilles insertion is in line with the distal Achilles. Proximally, the incision starts just medial to the Achilles and extends onto the calcaneus as distally as the surgeon needs to go (Fig. 18.9). As long as the incision is kept posterior, the nerve will be safe. Scissor dissection should be used proximally to isolate the plantaris tendon and to keep the dissection in the anterior posterior plane. The difficulty comes if the dissection drifts medially; the neurovascular bundle can then be damaged. Once safely on the bone, a subperiosteal dissection should be anterior, posterior, and lateral on the calcaneus, lifting the Achilles and the plantaris insertions up off the distal insertional ridge. An elevator can be used to expose the central and lateral portion of the calcaneus, and the retrocalcaneal bursa can be easily accessed from this incision. The FHL can be accessed, but the preferred approach for FHL harvest is the modification described below.

A useful variant of the medial approach is the medial approach with the lateral extension (Fig. 18.10).[2] This allows for a central splitting approach to the tendon pathology and a medial approach to the FHL. This also allows for the placement of drill holes or anchors in the central calcaneus in order to anchor the FHL transfer. The key to using this approach safely is to have a flap of tissue that exposes the distal Achilles, but that includes the Achilles peritenon

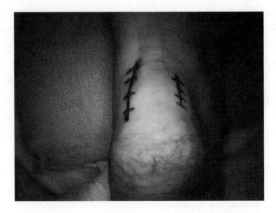

Fig. 18.9. Incision location for combined medial and lateral incisions

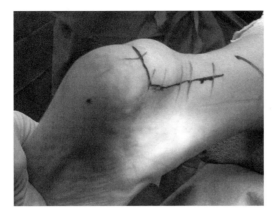

Fig. 18.10. Medial approach with lateral extension

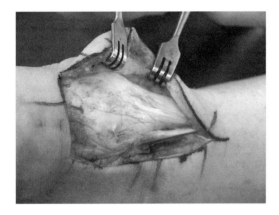

Fig. 18.11. Full-thickness peritenon flap

(Fig. 18.11). The distal medial to lateral extension incision needs to be in a normal posterior Achilles skin fold. The incision should be full thickness on the transverse portion until reaching the Achilles. The flap is carefully lifted up by sharply teasing the peritenon away from the Achilles. Limited retraction should be done at the 90-degree angle of the extension. The extension can extend all the way lateral until the sural nerve is encountered. The FHL is best approached deep to the most proximal portion of the Achilles that is exposed. Scissor dissection anterior to the central portion of the Achilles will expose the FHL muscle belly after going through the thin fascia to the deep posterior compartment (Fig. 18.12). The FHL tendon can be found by tracking the distal muscle belly to the tendon. From this incision, the FHL can be released into and through the FHL tunnel under the sustentaculum tali. At, and distal to, the musculotendinous junction of the FHL, the neurovascular bundle is directly medial to the tendon. The nerve and the artery need to be protected when the FHL tendon is harvested.

The lateral and medial approaches can be done at the same time (Fig. 18.9). The only caveat is that most surgeons limit the medial incision in length, and

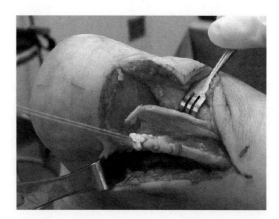

Fig. 18.12. Flexor hallucis longus (FHL) harvest through a medial approach with lateral extension

the skin bridge between the incisions should be maximized. There is no formal recommendation as to the size of the bridge.

Conclusion

The medial and lateral approaches to the distal Achilles are both versatile and functional. These approaches should be part of the Achilles surgeon's armamentarium.

References

1. Watson AD, Anderson RB, Davis WH. Comparison of results of retrocalcaneal decompression for retrocalcaneal bursitis and insertional Achilles tendinosis with calcific spur. Foot Ankle Int 2000;21(8):638.
2. Den Hartog B. Flexor hallicus longus transfer for chronic Achilles tendinosis. Foot Ankle Int 2003;24(3):233–7.
3. McGarvey WC, Palumbo RC, Baxter DE, et al. Insertional Achilles tendinosis: Surgical treatment through a central tendon splitting approach. Foot Ankle Int 2002;23(1):19–25.
4. Gerken P, McGarvey WC, Baxter DE. Insertional Achilles tendinitis. Foot Ankle Clin North Am 1996;112(1):237–48.
5. Chao W, Del JT, Bates JE, et al. Achilles tendon insertion: an in vitro anatomic study. Foot Ankle Int 1997;18(2):81–4.
6. Myerson M, et al. Mandelbaum B. Disorders of the Achilles tendon and retrocalcaneal region. In: Myerson M, ed. Foot and Ankle Disorders. Philadelphia: WB Saunders, 2000:1367–98.
7. Lagergren C, Lindholm A. Vascular distribution in the Achilles tendon: an angiographic and microangiographic study. Acta Chir Scand 1959;116:491.
8. Heneghan MA, Pavlov H. The Haglund painful heel syndrome: experimental investigation of cause and therapeutic implications. Clin Orthop Rel Res 1984;187:228–34.
9. Wapner KL, Pavlock GS, Hecht PJ. Repair of chronic Achilles tendon rupture with flexor hallucis longus tendon transfer. Foot Ankle Int 1993;14(8):443–9.

19

Insertional Achilles Tendinopathy: The Central Approach

James A. Nunley and John S. Reach, Jr.

Insertional Achilles tendinopathy is a painful, frequently disabling condition of the posterior foot and ankle. Discomfort and irritation typically arise along the posterior aspect of the heel. As with most tendinopathies, pain begins intermittently and gradually becomes constant as the disease progresses. A common sign of this insertional tendon disease is the patient's difficulty in wearing closed-back shoes. Athletically inclined patients may report more pain after exercise.

Despite advances in basic science tendon research, the pathophysiology of insertional Achilles tendinopathy is still not well understood. Traditionally, the disease has been viewed as an overuse phenomenon. Shear forces between collagen fascicles as well as biomechanical problems at the osseotendinous junction have been cited as causative factors in the disease. Recently, molecular collagen studies have hinted at the role of tenocytic chondral metaplasia as a causative factor.[1] Other studies have focused on the role of increased microcirculation at the point of pain in insertional tendinopathy.[2] It is not clear whether these findings represent etiologic or secondary factors.

Insertional Achilles tendinopathy manifests in two very different patient populations: young active athletes and older sedentary patients. In the former group, pain is related to athletic activity and overuse. Running, dancing, tennis, and basketball are associated sports that tend to involve repetitive jumping and vigorous push-off activities. Pain seldom affects activities of daily living in this patient population. Pain usually presents at the initiation of sports activities and again just following activities. These patients' symptoms may be aggravated by running on hard surfaces, uneven ground, or uphill. Patients almost invariably present in open-backed shoes or sandals. Generally, this group appears to do well with conservative treatment.

The latter group of patients is typically older than 45 years of age, sedentary, overweight, frequently female (although men can also be affected), and frequently have numerous medical comorbidities. Pain in these patients appears to be caused by degenerative changes rather than overuse. They, too, find open-backed shoes or sandals most comfortable. This group appears to do poorly with conservative treatment.

J.A. Nunley (ed.), *The Achilles Tendon: Treatment and Rehabilitation*,
DOI: 10.1007/978-1-387-79206-4_19, © Springer Science+Business Media, LLC 2009

On physical exam, an inflamed retrocalcaneal bursa or a posterolateral bony ridge may be noted. Tenderness is usually localized to the central lateral portion of the calcaneus at the tendon insertion. Pain is rarely found medially. The

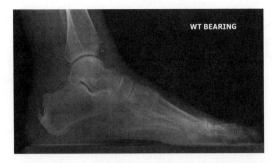

Fig.19.1. Lateral radiograph in the weight-bearing position demonstrating ossification within the Achilles tendon, as well as a sharp prominence to the posterior superior calcaneus

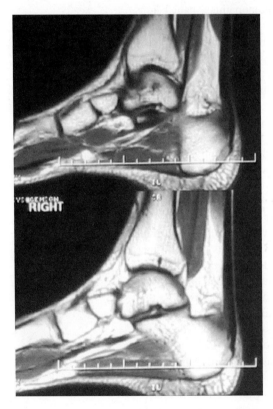

A

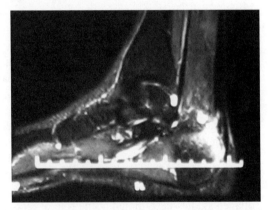

B

C

Fig. 19.2. Lateral magnetic resonance imaging (MRI) and ultrasound showing tendinopathy and calcifications (same patient as in Figure 19.1). (A) T1–weighted image demonstrates calcification within the Achilles tendon. (B) T2–weighted image shows bone edema changes within the posterior calcaneus and extensive bone edema changes within the posterior calcaneus. (C) Ultrasound image demonstrates calcification in the retrocalcaneal bursa

gastrocnemius-soleus complex may be tight with decreased ankle dorsiflexion when compared to the contralateral heel cord. Swelling and broadening of the heel is common. Crepitus and generalized erythema may also be observed. Pain is typically exacerbated by forced ankle dorsiflexion.

Plain x-ray studies often demonstrate Haglund's deformity as well as intra-tendinous bone spurs wisping back from the bone–tendon junction (Fig. 19.1). Both magnetic resonance imaging (MRI) and ultrasonography may demonstrate lakes of tendinopathy within fibers of healthy tendon (Fig. 19.2). Both of these soft tissue imaging modalities may offer an advantage in the preoperative planning of tendon debridement. Ultrasound imaging, particularly with color Doppler imaging, has proven to be a quite helpful in the authors' hands.

Differential Diagnosis

Insertional enthesopathy
Seronegative spondyloarthropathies
   Reactive arthritis (Reiter's syndrome)
   Ankylosing spondylitis
   Psoriatic arthritis
   Inflammatory disease of the bowel
      Crohn's disease
      Ulcerative colitis
Gout
Tendinosis of systemic corticosteroids
Tendinosis of quinolone antibiotics
Sarcoidosis
Diffuse idiopathic skeletal hyperostosis (DISH)
Infection
Positional (ridged heel counter, occupational)
Traumatic blow
Overuse tendinosis
"Pump bump"
Retrocalcaneal bursitis
Haglund disease
Sever's disease (apophysis closes by 15 years)

Case Study

A 63-year-old woman presented with a history of being troubled by tendonitis and bone spurs in her Achilles tendon for several years. She had been treated by her local podiatrist with physical therapy, heel lifts, immobilization, and one cortisone injection. She continued to have significant pain and felt that her tendon was in danger of rupturing. The patient specifically indicated that 5 months prior to her presentation to us, she had a marked increase in her heel pain.

Physical examination revealed a slightly obese female with a large protruding lump at the base of her left Achilles tendon. She was able to perform a double heel rise, but unable to perform a single heel rise. Her strength was recorded as normal and her ankle dorsiflexed slightly more than the opposite normal side.

Her plain radiographs showed a calcification within the Achilles tendon and large Haglund's deformity (posterior-superior calcaneal tuberosity). An MRI was obtained preoperatively to assess the status of the Achilles tendon. It showed marked thickening and increased signal in the distal Achilles tendon just proximal to the attachment, compatible with chronic tendinopathy and partial tear. Otherwise, the MRI was normal.

The patient was taken to surgery where she underwent excision of a 5 × 2 cm degenerative area of the Achilles tendon along with excision of the Haglund's deformity. This was done with the patient in the prone position, with a central midline Achilles tendon splitting incision. Three corkscrew anchors 3.5 mm in diameter were inserted into the flush-cut surface of the calcaneus on the medial and lateral sides for reattachment of the Achilles tendon.

Postoperatively, the patient was maintained in a splint in slight plantarflexion for 2 weeks, at which point her sutures were removed and her leg was placed in a walking cast with her foot at neutral.

At 5 weeks postoperatively, her cast was converted to a walking boot that was removable for range-of-motion exercises. Two months postoperatively she began using a walking shoe with a half-inch heel wedge and started doing gastrocnemius strengthening exercises. At 4 months postoperatively she had no pain and was able to perform double heel rises and could perform a single heel rise in the swimming pool.

Four years postoperatively, the patient returned for an unrelated problem with her great toe. At that time she had symmetrical calves, no recurrence of swelling in the distal Achilles tendon, normal strength and normal range of motion, and her radiographs showed no recurrent calcification.

Treatment

Nonoperative

Nonoperative treatment centers on activity modification, resting the tendon, antiinflammatory modalities, and symptomatic pain relief. In the younger athletic patient, nonimpact cross-training may be implemented: water running, elliptical training, cycling, and swimming. Exacerbating activities (hill running, high-mileage workouts, and running on hard surfaces) should be curtailed. Patients may decrease inflammation through the judicious use of an oral nonsteroidal antiinflammatory medication (keeping in mind the recent cardiac literature[19,20]), and by localized ice massage. Shoes may be modified to relieve direct and biomechanical stress on the Achilles tendon by the use of a small heel lift, a U-shaped Achilles pad, softer heel counters, or backless shoes. If the clinician finds evidence of aberrant lower extremity alignment, a semi-rigid orthosis may be considered.

A program of gentle physical therapy complements nonoperative care in the young athlete. Therapy should focus on hamstring and gastrocnemius-soleus flexibility. Others have advocated eccentric calf-muscle training.[3] Contrast baths, ultrasound,[4] and iontophoresis may help control pain and inflammation at the site of maximum discomfort. Others have experienced success with injection of sclerosing agents.[5] Finally, the use of a short weight-bearing leg cast may be used to facilitate tendon resting. It is clear from numerous studies that the clinician should avoid the injection of corticosteroids directly into the tendon due to an unacceptable rate of complications.[6]

Operative

Current surgical treatment includes debridement of the Achilles tendon insertion, and removal of the abnormal tendinosis tissue, osteophytes, intratendinous calcifications, and Haglund's deformity. A variety of surgical approaches have been described for the treatment of insertional Achilles tendinopathy: a medial J-shaped incision, a lateral incision, a combination of both medial and lateral incisions as well as the posterior midline central tendon splitting approach, and, ultimately, even complete detachment of the Achilles tendon with debridement followed by reinsertion. Medial and lateral approaches have been described to gain access to the Achilles tendon insertion, but may not permit adequate debridement of the Achilles tendon insertion. A central approach facilitates debridement, but may necessitate the detachment of the Achilles tendon from the calcaneus.

Authors' Preferred Method

We advocate attempting nonoperative treatment for a period of 6 months. If the symptoms persist after nonsurgical modalities have failed, operative intervention is indicated. Prior to surgery the risks, benefits, and expected 10- to 12-month recovery time is discussed with the patient in detail.

The patient undergoes appropriate anesthesia and has a thigh-high tourniquet placed and the leg exsanguinated while supine on the gurney. We have found that early placement of the tourniquet affords easier and less traumatic patient positioning. The patient is then positioned prone on the operating table. A central heel-splitting incision provides ideal exposure to the degenerative tendinosis, the ectopic calcification within the tendon, the retrocalcaneal bursitis, and the Haglund's deformity (Figure 19.3). Sharp dissection preserves

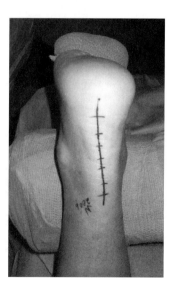

Fig. 19.3. Surgical incision plan. Patient is in the prone position, central midline split tendon splitting incision to be utilized

thick skin flaps. The paratendon is longitudinally incised and preserved for later closure.

It is essential to devote meticulous attention to the care of the wound edges throughout the procedure. Wound problems have been seen in all types of Achilles surgery. One must remember that the blood supply comes in medially and laterally. There is very little subcutaneous tissue overlying the distal Achilles tendon. We recommend sharp dissection and then judicious use of shin hooks. Tissue forceps should be avoided as should self-retaining retractors that stretch the skin. From the central approach, the Achilles tendon is divided over 6 to 10 cm. The pathologic process is easy to identify and treat by incising directly though the tendon's midline, coincident with the tendon fibers (Fig. 19.4). Once exposed, resection of the inflamed retrocalcaneal bursa, removal of the prominent posterolateral bone on the superior calcaneal ridge, and debridement of the calcific and diseased tendon insertion is performed with saw, osteotome, and rongeur (Fig. 19.5). We feel that an aggressive bony decompression results in improved patient satisfaction (Fig. 19.6) Adequacy of bony resection is confirmed by both direct visualization and intraoperative fluoroscopic lateral heel imaging (Fig. 19.7)

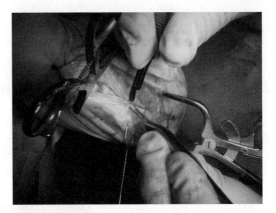

Fig. 19.4. The central split in the Achilles tendon

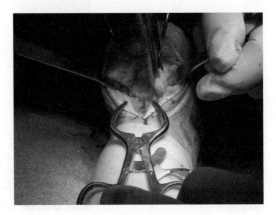

Fig. 19.5. Removal of bone and bursa from the superior calcaneal surface

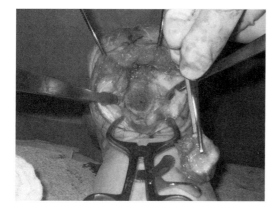

A

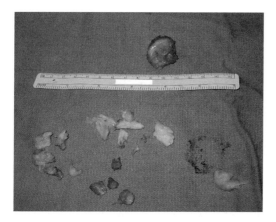

B

Fig. 19.6. (A) Resection of the entire Haglund's deformity. (B) Surgical specimen showing Haglund's deformity as well as degenerative tendon and ossification within the Achilles tendon

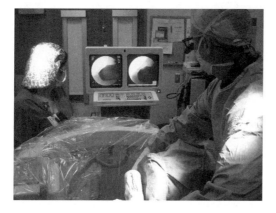

Fig. 19.7. Intraoperative fluoroscopy to demonstrate adequacy of bony resection

To facilitate an appropriate resection of bone and debridement of diseased tendon, a large proportion of the Achilles tendon may need to be detached. Our prior biomechanics study has determined that up to 50% of the insertion may be detached without rupture under three times body-weight load.[7] A subsequent clinical study of 52 heels found a low risk of subsequent avulsion if greater than 50% of the tendon was left intact.[8] Based on these studies, we recommend reattachment of the tendon with suture anchors directly to the calcaneus at the isometric point if greater than 50% of the insertion is detached (Fig. 19.8). In cases where the entire area of the insertion of the tendon is diseased, a prior study has found that plantarflexion strength is not altered after the complete detachment and reconstruction of the Achilles tendon with proximal V-Y lengthening and suture anchor reattachment.[9]

After adequate tendon debridement and bony resection, all bone edges are smoothed and feathered and bone fragments lavaged. The split Achilles fibers are reapproximated loosely with simple interrupted buried absorbable suture. The paratenon is reapproximated with a running absorbable stitch. We feel that closure of the paratenon is critical to prevent scar adherence of the skin to the Achilles tendon. The skin is closed with nonabsorbable monofilament vertical mattress stitch after a suction drain is placed (Fig. 19.9). The patient is placed in a non–weight bearing, bulky Robert-Jones dressing with the ankle in 10 degrees of plantarflexion.

Postoperatively, the dressing and sutures are removed at 2 weeks. The patient's leg is placed in a walking cast for an additional 2 weeks. Gentle range of motion is begun 4 weeks after surgery, and the patient may bear weight as tolerated in a removable walker boot. Unrestricted weight bearing is begun 8 weeks after surgery; however, the patient wears a half-inch heel lift for an additional 8 weeks. Plantarflexion strengthening is begun 10 to 12 weeks after surgery. Athletic activity is allowed at 6 months.

Complications of delayed wound healing, rupture of the Achilles tendon, and persistent insertional soreness have been reported. In the senior author's

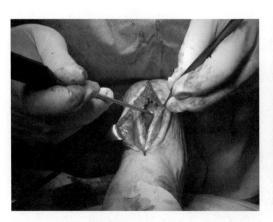
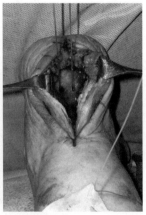

A   B

Fig. 19.8(A)   After completion of debridement, insertion of suture anchor for reattachment of distal portion of the Achilles tendon. (B) Two suture anchors into the calcaneus in preparation for securing distal Achilles tendon

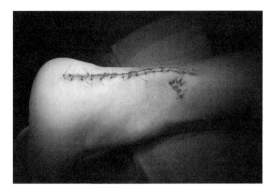

Fig. 19.9. Completed procedure with wound closed prior to splinting

personal series, 20 patients who were a minimum of 18 weeks postoperative returned for Cybex muscle testing and examination. Strength was equal to or greater on the operative side when compared to the nonoperative side. If revision surgery is required, one should consider the addition of a flexor hallucis longus (FHL) tendon transfer to augment the repair.

Results

Operative management of insertional calcific Achilles tendinopathy has been shown to be successful in most patients and satisfactory results have been reported in the literature ranging from 67% to 82%. Schepsis et al.[10,11] have recommended the use of a medial J-incision for both Achilles tendinitis as well as insertional tendinopathy. In their series of 45 surgical cases, of which all but two were competitive long distance runners, there were 24 cases of Achilles tendinitis, 14 cases of isolated retrocalcaneal bursitis, and seven patients who had signs and symptoms of both disorders. At a mean follow-up of 3 years there was an overall 87% satisfactory rate; however, 92% of the patients who had involvement of only the tendon yielded a satisfactory result, compared with only 71% satisfactory results in those patients who had retrocalcaneal bursitis. Interestingly, there were no reported skin complications.

The lateral surgical approach has been favored by Paavola et al.,[12] Watson et al.,[13] and Yodlowski et al.[14] In Yodlowski et al.'s series of 35 patients with 41 feet, utilizing a lateral incision it was possible to excise the diseased Achilles tendon and the retrocalcaneal bursa, and a partial calcaneal exostectomy was performed. At a 20-month follow-up, 90% of the patients had complete or significant relief, and 10% felt that they were improved. There was one patient who had bothersome pain at the incision site, but there were no reported wound breakdowns. Paavola et al. also utilized the lateral incision in 50 patients, and at final follow-up 28 of the 42 (67%) were fully restored to physical activity and 35 patients (83% were asymptomatic). There were eight complications in the 42 patients (19%), of which four were superficial wound infections, two were skin edge necrosis, and two were fibrotic scar reactions or scar formations. Watson et al. reported on 38 feet treated with a lateral approach and complications occurred in eight, or 21 %, of the series. One patient had avulsion of the Achilles tendon from its insertion and a second foot required reoperation for symptomatic radiographic recurrence. In addition, three feet developed symptoms of sural neuritis, and three feet had persistent hyperesthesia of the surgical scar. Watson et al. did not report any wound healing complications.

In 1992, Clain and Baxter[15] recommended the two-incision technique, which entails an incision both on the medial and on the lateral side of the Achilles tendon. The first incision is made on the symptomatic side where the maximum tenderness is. From this incision the Haglund's deformity is aggressively resected, as is the chronically inflamed retrocalcaneal bursa. There are no statistics quoted in this review article and no mention of complications.

In 1988, Kleiger[16] recommended starting the dissection laterally, parallel to the Achilles tendon with resection of the Haglund's deformity and retrocalcaneal bursa. When the bursal sac is large and projects medially, he recommended making a similar "medial perotendinous incision." This allows the surgeon to retract the posterior tibial neurovascular bundle and to further excise any degenerative tendon. His article does not discuss complications or patient series.

The posterior midline central tendon splitting incision was first described by McGarvey et al.[17] and Clain and Baxter,[15] and more recently by Johnson et al.[18] In Johnson et al.'s series of 22 patients followed for an average of 34 months, pain was significantly decreased, and function was improved. In their series, 55% of the patients preoperatively were unable to work full time and this was reduced to 9% postoperatively. The authors reported no neurovascular complications in two cases of superficial partial wound dehiscence that required dressing changes. No recurrence of calcific tendinopathy occurred, and there were no Achilles tendon ruptures. This would mirrors our results, in which 100% of the patients followed for a minimum of 2 years were completely satisfied, and with isokinetic testing were actually stronger on the operative side than on the nonoperative side. All authors utilizing the central approach have noted that it requires 11 to 12 months postoperatively for patients to reach their maximum potential in terms of both pain reduction and strength.

References

1. Maffulli N, Reaper J, Ewen SW, et al. Chondral metaplasia in calcific insertional tendinopathy of the Achilles tendon. Clin J Sport Med 2006;16(4):329–34.
2. Knobloch K, Kraemer R, Lichtenberg A, et al. Achilles tendon and paratendon microcirculation in midportion and insertional tendinopathy in athletes. Am J Sports Med 2006;34(1):92–7.
3. Fahlstrom M, Jonsson P, Lorentzon R, et al. Chronic Achilles tendon pain treated with eccentric calf-muscle training. Knee Surg Sports Traumatol Arthrosc 2003;11(5):327–33.
4. Furia JP. High-energy extracorporeal shock wave therapy as a treatment for insertional Achilles tendinopathy. Am J Sports Med 2006;34(5):733–40.
5. Ohberg L, Alfredson H. Sclerosing therapy in chronic Achilles tendon insertional pain-results of a pilot study. Knee Surg Sports Traumatol Arthrosc 2003;11(5):339–43.
6. Scutt N, Rolf C, Scutt A. Glucocorticoids inhibit tenocyte proliferation and tendon progenitor cell recruitment. J Orthop Res 2006;24(2):173–82.

7. Kolodziej P, Glisson RR, Nunley JA. Risk of avulsion of the Achilles tendon after partial excision for treatment of insertional tendonitis and Haglund's deformity: a biomechanical study. Foot Ankle Int 1999;20(7):433–7.

8. Calder JD, Saxby TS. Surgical treatment of insertional Achilles tendinosis. Foot Ankle Int 2003;24(2):119–21.

9. Wagner E, Gould J, Bilen E, et al. Change in plantarflexion strength after complete detachment and reconstruction of the Achilles tendon. Foot Ankle Int 2004;25(11):800–4.

10. Schepsis AA, Jones H, Haas AL. Achilles tendon disorders in athletes. Am J Sports Med 2002;30(2):287–305.

11. Schepsis AA, Wagner C, Leach RE. Surgical management of Achilles tendon overuse injuries. A long-term follow-up study. Am J Sports Med 1994;22(5):611–9.

12. Paavola M, Kannus P, Paakkala T, et al. Long-term prognosis of patients with Achilles tendinopathy. Am J Sports Med 2000;28(5):634–42.

13. Watson AD, Anderson RB, Davis WH. Comparison of results of retrocalcaneal decompression for retrocalcaneal bursitis and insertional Achilles tendinosis with calcific spur. Foot Ankle Int 2000;21(8):638–42.

14. Yodlowski ML, Scheller AD Jr, Minos L. Surgical treatment of Achilles tendinitis by decompression of the retrocalcaneal bursa and the superior calcaneal tuberosity. Am J Sports Med 2002;30(3):318–21.

15. Clain MR, Baxter DE. Achilles tendinitis. Foot Ankle 1992;13(8):482–7.

16. Kleiger, B. The posterior calcaneal tubercle impingement syndrome. Orthop Rev 1988;17(5):487–93.

17. McGarvey WC, Palumbo RC, Baxter DE, et al. Insertional Achilles tendinosis: surgical treatment through a central tendon splitting approach. Foot Ankle Int 2002;23(1):19–25.

18. Johnson KW, Zalavras C, Thordarson DB. Surgical management of insertional calcific Achilles tendinosis with a central tendon splitting approach. Foot Ankle Int 2006;27(4):245–50.

19. Graham DJ COX-2 inhibitors, other NSAIDs, and cardiovascular risk: the seduction of common Sense. JAMA. 2006;296(13): 1653–6. Epub 2006 Sep 1

20. Hernández-Diaz S, Varas-Lorenzo C, García Rodríguez LA Non-steroidal anti-inflammatory drugs and the risk of acute myocardial infarction. Basic Clin Pharmacol Toxicol. 2006;98(3):266–74.

20

Treatment of Chronic Achilles Tendon Ruptures with an Acellular Dermal Matrix Augmentation

Troy S. Watson and James A. Nunley

Although Achilles tendon repairs have been augmented using fascia lata, gastrocnemius flaps, plantaris tendon grafts, the palmaris longus, the flexor hallucis longus, and synthetic grafts,[1–7] the implementation of a single surgical model has not been universally accepted. Some studies reporting marginal improvement or equivalent results between direct repair and augmentation concluded that any advantages with augmentation did not merit the additional surgical risks in acute Achilles tendon repair.[2,8] In chronic Achilles tendon tears, however, the use of augmentation with primary repair or transfers has received greater acceptance. The reinforcement of chronic or neglected Achilles tear repairs is logically advantageous due to the poor tendon tissue quality present, the gap that remains following excision of the fibrous pseudotendon, and the tendon retraction or fatty infiltration resulting from delayed treatment.[9–14] Patients with chronic Achilles tendon ruptures are more technically challenging than those with acute ruptures; they have slower return to activity, higher complication rates, and greater functional deficits than their acute counterparts.[2,11–13,15] Although the idea of reinforcing chronic tears is generally accepted, the method for supporting the primary repair is not standardized. Unfortunately, many of the augmentation techniques in current use require the harvest of a healthy, autogenous tendon. Although these techniques have been shown to benefit the patient, the sacrifice of autologous tendons can be of concern since these tendons may be inadequate in length or diameter for Achilles repair.[5,16] If local tendons are rerouted or removed, the biomechanical and soft tissue effects on the foot should also be taken into consideration.[6,11,14,17] Misgivings regarding the use of local tendons or a lack of suitable tendons in specific patients has spurred the investigation of allografts and synthetic materials as a means of Achilles augmentation. Synthetic materials have offered good results[1]; however, since such materials do not incorporate or facilitate tendon regeneration over time, they merely offer interim strength, which may ultimately cause problems.[9]

J.A. Nunley (ed.), *The Achilles Tendon: Treatment and Rehabilitation*,
DOI: 10.1007/978-1-387-79206-4_20, © Springer Science+Business Media, LLC 2009

Recently, the use of an acellular human dermal matrix has received attention as a material for augmenting chronic Achilles tendon injuries. An allograft in sheet form allows the surgeon to reinforce a tendon repair without sacrificing local tissues. Ideally, the reinforcing material offers additional stability to the repair, facilitates cellular infiltration without inflammation, and incorporates into the tendon over time. In a study by Lee,[18] nine neglected Achilles tendon ruptures were augmented with an acellular tissue graft and followed for a minimum of 20 months. There were no reruptures or instances of recurrent pain within this group. The patients had an average return-to-activity time of 15.2 weeks and an average American Orthopedic Association of Foot and Ankle Surgeons (AOFAS) ankle hindfoot score of 86.2 at 12 months. The return to activity time in this series was markedly faster than previous reports in chronic ruptures treated with primary repair alone or with turndown flaps. These positive results were particularly interesting since the majority of the treated patients had comorbidities of smoking or diabetes. In a technique study by Brigido et al.,[19] 21 Achilles tendons were treated with the acellular dermal matrix for chronic Achilles tendinosis when greater than 50% of the tendon was excised due to disease. In that population, patients returned to activity at an average of 12.1 weeks after surgery.

Collectively, these clinical results correspond to the preclinical performance of this extracellular matrix in cellular studies, animal models, and biomechanical testing. Mechanical testing of a variety of extracellular matrices by Barber et al.[20] showed that the suture pullout strength was higher (157 to 229 N) for this type of material than all other materials tested. The inherent mechanical properties and suture purchase offered by the matrix should aid in the intraoperative and preliminary postoperative reinforcement of the primary repair prior to graft incorporation. The initial strength properties of an acellular dermal matrix construct were also statistically equivalent to palmaris longus tendon grafts in a biomechanical study of medial collateral ligament elbow reconstruction.[21] This acellular human dermal graft has repeatedly reflected regenerative tissue properties, a lack of inflammation, and cellular incorporation in a variety of canine, porcine, and rat models as well as in vitro cellular testing.[22–26] The incorporation and regenerative nature of the acellular human dermal matrix is attributed to processing methods maintaining an intact native connective tissue structure rather than damaging or cross-linking the matrix.[23] The augmentation of rotator cuff tendinous tissue with this material has been accomplished successfully and provided reduced re-tear rates and good functional outcomes clinically using a number of different techniques.[27–30] Anecdotal evidence indicates that the positive histology reports with this material in preclinical models correspond to the clinical cellular response seen in patients. In postoperative graft biopsies of the rotator cuff, there was notable formation of a neotendon populated by healthy cells and blood vessels.[30]

Treatment

In comparison to the primary Achilles tendon rupture, options for the neglected cases can present challenges for even the experienced foot and ankle surgeon. Treatment options include conservative measures for those in whom surgical intervention may be contraindicated and surgery for those with functional deficits that would benefit from repair.

Nonoperative treatment is indicated in patients who are low demand or who have a significant contraindication to surgical intervention. Patients with comorbidities, such as significant cardiac disease, peripheral vascular disease, or other systemic problems, may be best treated nonoperatively. Patients should be evaluated thoroughly and their demands and activity level reviewed. Consultation with a primary care provider can be helpful in difficult cases. Options for these patients include use of a CAM walker boot for 2 to 3 months or placement of an ankle-foot orthosis to aid walking. Patients should understand that despite the above modalities, they will likely continue to walk with an antalgic gait.

The decision of which surgical technique to employ is largely predicated on the gap that remains after the fibrous tissue is resected from the tendon. Gaps of 1 to 2 cm can usually be reapproximated with blunt dissection between the superficial and deep compartments of the lower leg and manual traction of the proximal portion of the Achilles tendon. A suture weave placed in the proximal portion of the Achilles is used to pull manual distraction distally until the gap is closed. An end-to-end anastomosis of the Achilles is then completed utilizing a two-strand technique.

For gaps larger than 2 cm and up to 6 cm, a V-Y lengthening procedure can be added to the procedure described above. Abraham and Pankovich 10 described a technique in which an inverted V incision is made proximally in the fascia, manual distraction directed distally until an end-to-end anastomosis is achieved, and the resultant inverted Y is then repaired. This is discussed in detail in Chapter 10.

Larger gaps that cannot be adequately spanned with the above techniques may require use of tendon transfer procedures. Stretching of the Achilles muscle tendon unit greater than 5 to 6 cm may compromise the strength of this structure, and most clinicians would recommend other means of spanning gaps of this size.[31] In a recently published study, Elias et al.[32] reported on 15 cases of neglected Achilles tendon rupture undergoing reconstruction using a V-Y lengthening combined with a flexor hallucis longus (FHL) tendon transfer through a single incision. Den Hartog[33] published his series of patients treated with a single incision with transfer of the FHL for chronic pathology of the Achilles tendon. As an alternative to the one-incision technique, others have advocated a transfer of the FHL[34,35] or flexor digitorum longus (FDL)[36] through a two-incision technique. In these techniques, the transferred tendon with its additional length is used to span the gap, rather than the use of V-Y lengthening. These techniques are described in more detail in Chapter 11.

As an adjunct to the above procedures, and as a possible way of completely avoiding a tendon transfer procedure, an acellular dermal matrix has been used in conjunction with gastrocnemius lengthening to achieve repair of the chronically ruptured Achilles tendon.[18,19,37] This technique has been used in cases where the tendon gap measures up to 6 cm in length. In gaps larger than this, a single-incision technique is utilized with harvest of the FHL tendon in its tunnel as it courses around the medial ankle. The FHL tendon is then fixed to the calcaneus with a biosorb interference screw. This technique is described as well in Chapter 11. Augmentation with the acellular dermal matrix in these cases can be included to add structural integrity to the repair.

The procedure for treatment of the chronic Achilles tendon rupture is begun by placing the patient in the prone position with all bony prominences padded

(Fig. 20.1). A thigh tourniquet is used for these procedures. A preoperative popliteal block will aid in postoperative pain control.

A long incision is made over the posteromedial leg extending from the musculotendinous junction of the gastrocnemius to theinsertion of the Achilles tendon in the calcaneus. The incision is placed medially to avoid injury to the sural nerve, but then curves more centrally over the proximal portion to allow for exposure for the V-Y lengthening. Full-thickness skin flaps are developed with the paratenon over the Achilles, longitudinally incised for later closure. The fibrous portion of the Achilles tendon is identified (Fig. 20.2).and is carefully excised until more organized tendon fibers are encountered. At this point, the size of the gap is measured intraoperatively and the decisions for reconstructive technique are made. As stated previously, for gaps up to 5 to 6 cm, a proximal V-Y lengthening is performed in an attempt to gain tendon length and bridge the gap (Fig. 20.3). A suture weave is placed after the inverted V cut is made in the gastrocnemius fascia. The suture weave is started proximally with a No. 2 Fiberwire (Arthrex, Inc., Naples, FL) just distal to the inverted V. A second strand of Fiberwire is placed starting 3 to 4 cm distal

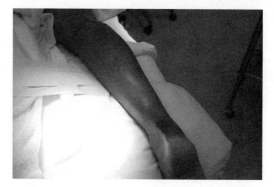

Fig. 20.1. Prone positioning. For the chronic rupture, the contralateral extremity is not prepped for comparison

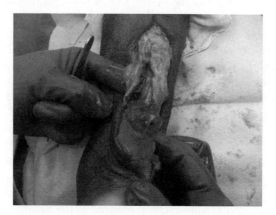

Fig. 20.2. Elevation of full-thickness skin flaps reveals a disorganized, fibrous scar or pseudotendon

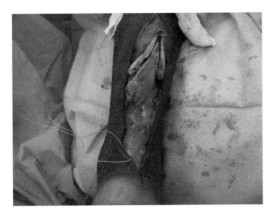

Fig. 20.3. V-Y lengthening of gastrocnemius with manual traction being applied

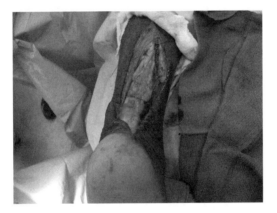

Fig. 20.4. Fixation of end-to-end anastomosis with two-stranded technique

to the gap and brought proximally. Using manual traction for 3 to 5 minutes, stretching of the proximal limb is possible, making end-to-end anastomosis possible. With an assistant holding the two ends of the tendon together, the two medial strands and two lateral strands are tied down (Fig. 20.4).

Attention is then turned to the repair of the V-Y lengthening. This is typically completed with 2-0 absorbable suture (Fig. 20.5). In cases where the gap cannot be closed or in cases where additional augmentation is warranted, an FHL tendon harvest can be completed and fixed to the calcaneus with a biotenodesis screw.

With the primary repair completed, including the gastrocnemius lengthening, attention is turned to placement of the acellular dermal matrix. Standard and thick versions of the acellular human dermal matrix (Graftjacket® Matrix, Wright Medical Technology, Inc., Arlington, TN) can be utilized (Fig. 20.6). Typically, the standard thickness is easier to manipulate and fashion to the Achilles tendon. The graft can be used as either an onlay graft or a wrap. Most often, the graft is wrapped around the tendon forming a complete cylinder (Fig. 20.7). The graft is sutured down the seam after trimming away redundant

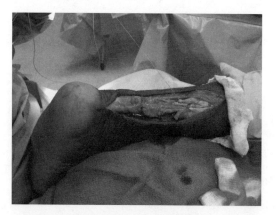

Fig. 20.5. Repair of the V-Y gastrocnemius lengthening using absorbable suture

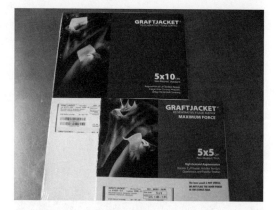

Fig. 20.6. Two forms of acellular dermal matrix available: standard and thick

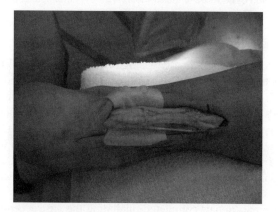

Fig. 20.7. Acellular dermal matrix wrap technique

material (Fig. 20.8). This seam is then rotated for anterior placement and the Graftjacket Matrix is sutured to the tendon with 2-0 Vicryl suture to ensure good fixation and graft to native tendon contact (Fig. 20.9). The wound is closed without tension using a layered closure (Fig. 20.10). A splint is applied

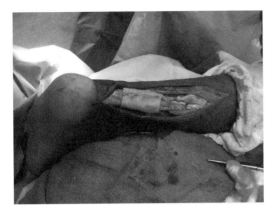

Fig. 20.8. After wrapping of the acellular dermal matrix, suture of the seam is completed. It is important not to suture the graft to the Achilles tendon at this point

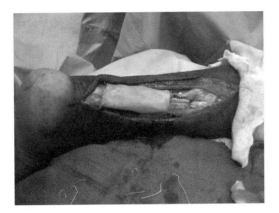

Fig. 20.9. The acellular dermal matrix is then rotated 180 degrees and sutured down to the Achilles tendon using absorbable suture. Care is taken to secure the graft to the tendon with multiple sutures to prevent postsurgical delamination of the graft

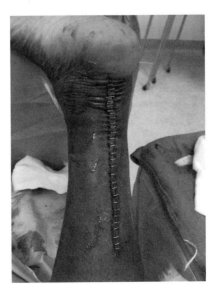

Fig. 20.10. Closure without tension of the posterior wound before application of a splint

to the limb with the foot in a plantarflexed position to avoid stress on the repair. The patient is given a cold therapy unit in the recovery room and is discharged.

Case Study 1: Chronic Achilles Rupture

A 28-year-old policewoman injured her right ankle while boxing 3 months prior to presentation in the office. She was pursuing a career as a professional fighter at the time of injury. After reporting to the emergency room, she was diagnosed with a severe ankle sprain and placed into a stirrup ankle brace. At 6 weeks postinjury, she attempted to return to boxing, noting both pain and lack of push-off strength with her right lower extremity. She sought medical attention under her primary care physician who sent her to physical therapy for her ankle sprain. With no notable improvement at 3 months postinjury, she was referred to an orthopedic surgeon.

Upon presentation, the patient was noted to walk with an antalgic gait. Physical exam found no lateral ankle instability and no tenderness over the anterotalofibular ligament, but the patient had a positive Thompson test with an atrophied calf muscle belly. The patient was sent for an magnetic resonance imaging (MRI), as no palpable defect was evident in the Achilles tendon. Review of the MRI revealed a chronic rupture with fibrosis and thickening over a large segment of the tendon.

Given the patient's age, occupation, and desire for a professional boxing career, surgical intervention was offered to restore functionality to the Achilles tendon and attempt to return the patient to preinjury performance levels. After informed consent was obtained, the patient was placed on the schedule for operative intervention.

Intraoperative examination of the tendon revealed a region of disorganized fibers and intervening fibrous tissue (Fig. 20.11). Debridement was begun in this area and continued proximally and distally until normal tendon was encountered. A gap of 6 cm remained. Following this, a V-Y lengthening with end-to-end anastomosis was performed, followed be closure of the proximal Y. A standard thickness acellular human dermal matrix (Graftjacket Matrix) was then sutured over the direct repair of the Achilles as well as over the Y repair to augment and add strength to the construct (Fig. 20.12). The leg was

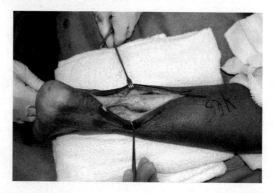

Fig. 20.11. Exposure reveals pseudotendon with scarring and fibrosis

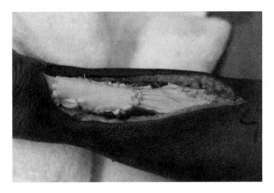

Fig. 20.12. Technique of onlay placement of the acellular dermal matrix

splinted in 15 degrees of plantarflexion, and local anesthesia was injected prior to leaving the operating room.

The patient was splinted for the first 2 weeks postoperatively, followed by the use of a CAM walker boot after the first follow-up visit. Non–weight bearing was continued for 6 weeks; however, the patient was allowed to work on active dorsiflexion and plantarflexion between weeks 2 and 6. At 6 weeks postoperatively, the patient was allowed to begin weight bearing in the boot. Formal physical therapy was begun at 8 weeks, and the boot was discontinued at 12 weeks postoperatively. Physical therapy continued until month 5, when the patient transitioned her recovery to the gym with a home strengthening program. At 10 months postsurgery, she returned to the ring and no longer had push-off weakness or other complaints related to the limb.

Case Study 2: Chronic Achilles Tendon Rupture

A 42-year-old construction worker was seen in the office following an injury that he incurred while playing basketball 4 months prior. He had been trying to work, but was experiencing increasing difficulty with the physical demands of his job.

His primary care provider had examined him once; however, the diagnosis was simply an ankle sprain that was not improving. He complained of walking with a limp, lack of strength when climbing a ladder, and pain over the posterior ankle region.

At the time of presentation, he was noted to walk with a slight limp, was unable to perform a single limb toe raise, and had a positive Thompson test. A defect was palpable over the Achilles tendon, approximately 3 to 4 cm from its attachment into the calcaneus. A chronic Achilles tendon tear diagnosis was made, and treatment options were discussed. After consenting to surgical intervention, an MRI was ordered to help determine the size of the gap in the tendon for preoperative planning (Fig. 20.13).

Intraoperatively the tendon was debrided of all fibrous tissue, leaving a gap of approximately 5 cm (Fig. 20.14). A V-Y gastrocnemius lengthening was then performed and a suture weave was placed into the proximal and distal ends of the debrided tendon using No. 2 Fiberwire (Fig. 20.15). Once an end-to-end anastomosis of the Achilles tendon was achieved, the strands of

Fig. 20.13 Magnetic resonance imaging (MRI) showing tendon gap and retraction of proximal limb

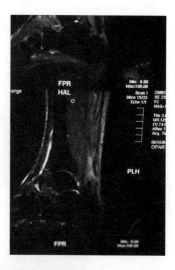

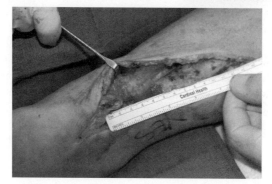

Fig. 20.14. Tendon gap as measured after debridement of fibrous tissue and scar

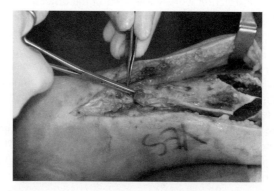

Fig. 20.15. V-Y lengthening with an assistant holding ends of the tendon together. Suture weave was performed next to secure the repair

Fiberwire were tied down with the foot held in about 20 degrees of plantar-flexion. The proximal V-Y was repaired with 2-0 nonabsorbable suture (Fig. 20.16). Having completed the repair, augmentation was achieved with a standard thickness 5- × 10-cm acellular dermal matrix graft (Graftjacket Matrix)

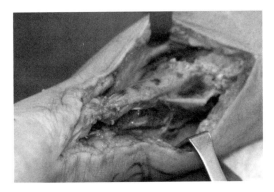

Fig. 20.16. End-to-end anastomosis of Achilles tendon and proximal repair of V-Y completed

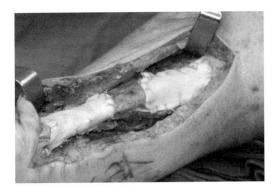

Fig. 20.17. Onlay placement of acellular dermal matrix at both proximal and distal repair sites

(Fig. 20.17). A standard layered closure was completed, and the patient was placed in a bulky dressing with a rigid splint in 15 degrees of plantarflexion.

Postoperative rehabilitation followed a similar protocol to that previously described in Case Study 1. At 5 months postsurgery, the patient returned to work. He avoided ladder climbing and working at height until 8 months after surgery. By month 10, he was able to perform a single limb toe raise.

References

1. Fernandez-Fairen M, et al. Gimeno C. Augmented repair of Achilles tendon ruptures. Am J Sports Med 1997;25:177–81.
2. Nyyssonen T, Saarikoski H, Kaukonen JP, et al. Simple end-to-end suture versus augmented repair in acute Achilles tendon ruptures: a retrospective comparison in 98 patients. Acta Orthop Scand 2003;74:206–8.
3. Lynn TA. Repair of the torn Achilles tendon, using the plantaris tendon as a reinforcing membrane. J Bone Joint Surg [Am] 1966;48:268–72.
4. Lindholm A. A new method of operation in subcutaneous rupture of the Achilles tendon. Acta Chir Scand 1959;117:261–70.
5. Pearsall AW, Bryant GK. Technique tip: a new technique for augmentation of repair of chronic Achilles tendon rupture. Foot Ankle Int 2006;27:146–7.

6. Miskulin M, Miskulin A, Klobucar H, et al. Neglected rupture of the Achilles tendon treated with peroneus brevis transfer: a functional assessment of 5 cases. J Foot Ankle Surg 2005;44:49–56.

7. Zell RA, Santoro VM. Augmented repair of acute Achilles tendon ruptures. Foot Ankle Int 2000;21:469–74.

8. Aktas S, Kocaoglu B, Nalbantoglu U, et al. End-to-end versus augmented repair in the treatment of acute Achilles tendon ruptures. J Foot Ankle Surg 2007;46:336–40.

9. Kissel CG, Blacklidge DK, Crowley DL. Repair of neglected Achilles tendon ruptures—procedure and functional results. J Foot Ankle Surg 1994;33:46–52.

10. Abraham E, Pankovich AM. Neglected rupture of the Achilles tendon. Treatment by V-Y tendinous flap. J Bone Joint Surg Am 1975;57:253–5.

11. Maffulli N, Leadbetter WB. Free gracilis tendon graft in neglected tears of the Achilles tendon. Clin J Sports Med 2005;15:56–61.

12. Pintore E, Barra V, Pintore R, et al. Peroneus brevis tendon transfer in neglected tears of the Achilles tendon. J Trauma 2001;50:71–8.

13. Gabel S, Manoli A 2nd. Neglected rupture of the Achilles tendon. Foot Ankle 1994; Int15:512–7.

14. Leppilahti J, Orava S. Total Achilles tendon rupture. A review. Sports Med 1998;25:79–100.

15. Saxena A, Cheung S. Surgery for chronic Achilles tendinopathy. Review of 91 procedures over 10 years. J Am Podiatr Med Assoc 2003;93:283–91.

16. Lee YS, Lin CC, Chen CN, et al. Reconstruction for neglected Achilles tendon rupture: the modified Bosworth technique. Orthopedics 2005;28:647–50.

17. Hahn F, Maiwald C, Horstmann T, et al. Changes in plantar pressure distribution after Achilles tendon augmentation with flexor hallucis longus transfer. Clin Biomech (Bristol, Avon) 2007.

18. Lee DK. Achilles tendon repair with acellular tissue graft augmentation in neglected ruptures. J Foot Ankle Surg 2007;46:451–5.

19. Brigido SA, Schwartz E, Barnett L, et al. Reconstruction of the diseased Achilles tendon using an acellular human dermal graft followed by early mobilization—a preliminary series. Tech Foot Ankle Surg 2007;6:249–53.

20. Barber FA, Herbert MA, Coons DA. Tendon augmentation grafts: biomechanical failure loads and failure patterns. Arthroscopy 2006;22:534–8.

21. Furukawa K, Pichora J, Steinmann S, et al. Efficacy of interference screw and double-docking methods using palmaris longus and GraftJacket for medial collateral ligament reconstruction of the elbow. J Shoulder Elbow Surg/Am Shoulder Elbow Surg 2007;16:449–53.

22. Beniker D, McQuillan D, Livesey S, et al. The use of acellular dermal matrix as a scaffold for periosteum replacement. Orthopedics 2003;26:s591–6.

23. Harper J, McQuillan D. A novel regenerative tissue matrix (RTM) technology for connective tissue reconstruction. Wounds 2007;19:163–8.

24. Valentin JE, Badylak JS, McCabe GP, et al. Extracellular matrix bioscaffolds for orthopaedic applications. A comparative histologic study. J Bone Joint Surg [Am] 2006:88:2673–86.

25. Adams JE, Zobitz ME, Reach JS Jr, et al. Rotator cuff repair using an acellular dermal matrix graft: an in vivo study in a canine model. Arthroscopy 2006;22:700–9.

26. Fini M, Torricelli P, Giavaresi G, et al. In vitro study comparing two collagenous membranes in view of their clinical application for rotator cuff tendon regeneration. J Orthop Res 2007;25:98–107.

27. Labbe MR. Arthroscopic technique for patch augmentation of rotator cuff repairs. Arthroscopy 2006;22:e1131–6.

28. Dopirak R, Bond J, Snyder S. Arthroscopic total rotator cuff replacement with an acellular human dermal allograft matrix. Int J shoulder Surg 2007;1:7–15.

29. Burkhead W, Schiffern S, Krishnan S. Use of Graft Jacket as an augmentation for massive rotator cuff tears. Semin Arthrosc 2007;18:11–18.
30. Snyder S, Bond J. Technique for arthroscopic replacement of severely damaged rotator cuff using "Graftjacket" allograft. Oper Tech Sports Med 2007;15:86–94.
31. Myerson MS. Achilles tendon ruptures. Instr Course Lectures 1999;48:219–30.
32. Elias I, Besser M, Nazarian LN, et al. Reconstruction for missed or neglected Achilles tendon ruptures with V-Y lengthening and flexor hallucis longus tendon transfer through one incision. Foot Ankle Int 2007;28:1238–48.
33. Den Hartog B. Flexor hallucis longus transfer for chronic Achilles tendinosus. Foot Ankle Int 2003;24:233–7.
34. Wapner KL, Pavlock GS, Hecht PJ, et al. Repair of chronic Achilles tendon rupture with flexor hallucis longus tendon transfer. Foot Ankle 1993;14:443–9.
35. Wapner KL, Hecht PJ. Repair of chronic Achilles tendon rupture with flexor hallucis longus tendon transfer. Oper Tech Orthop 1994;4:132–7.
36. Mann RA, Holmes GB Jr, Seale KS, et al. Chronic rupture of the Achilles tendon: a new technique of repair. J Bone Joint Surg [Am] 1991;73:214–9.
37. Lee MS. GraftJacket augmentation of chronic Achilles tendon ruptures. Orthopedics 2004;27:s151–3.

Index

Printed in the United States of America